Herbal Remedies & Natural Medicine Bible

A Practical Guide to Taking Care of Your Healing Herbs and Plants to Prepare Tinctures, Essential Oils, Infusions, and Microbicide Preparations.

JOANA GREEN

© Copyright 2023 by Joana Green - All rights reserved.

This document is geared towards providing exact and reliable information in regard to the topic and issue covered.

- From a Declaration of Principles which was accepted and approved equally by a Committee of the American Bar Association and a Committee of Publishers and Associations.

In no way is it legal to reproduce, duplicate, or transmit any part of this document in either electronic means or in printed format. All rights reserved.

The information provided herein is stated to be truthful and consistent, in that any liability, in terms of inattention or otherwise, by any usage or abuse of any policies, processes, or directions contained within is the solitary and utter responsibility of the recipient reader.

Under no circumstances will any legal responsibility or blame be held against the publisher for any reparation, damages, or monetary loss due to the information herein, either directly or indirectly. Respective authors own all copyrights not held by the publisher.

The information herein is offered for informational purposes solely and is universal as so. The presentation of the informaation is without contract or any type of guarantee assurance.

The trademarks that are used are without any consent, and the publication of the trademark is without permission or backing by the trademark owner. All trademarks and brands within this book are for clarifying purposes only and are owned by the owners themselves, not affiliated with this document.

Contents

INTRODUCTION

The world of natural medicine is vast and complex, filled with many herbs, plants, and remedies that have been used for centuries to promote healing and wellness. With so much information out there, it can be overwhelming to know where to start. That's where the Herbal Remedies Natural Medicine Bible comes in. This comprehensive guide provides readers with everything they need to know about the world of herbal remedies, including the history and uses of various herbs and plants, how to grow and harvest them, and how to prepare tinctures, essential oils, infusions, and antibiotics.

In this 5-in-1 guide, readers will learn about the healing properties of herbs and plants such as chamomile, lavender, and echinacea, as well as more obscure remedies like black cohosh and astragalus. With step-by-step instructions and detailed illustrations, even those new to natural medicine can feel confident in their ability to create herbal remedies.

In today's fast-paced world, where we are always on the go, maintaining a healthy lifestyle cannot be easy. Many of us rely on medications to treat common ailments, but did you know that herbal remedies have been used for centuries to treat a wide range of health issues? The Herbal Remedies Natural Medicine Bible: [5 in 1] The Practical Guide of Healing Herbs and Plants to Grow and Use for Preparing Tinctures, Essential Oils, Infusions, and Antibiotics is an essential guide for anyone interested in natural medicine.

This comprehensive guide covers everything from growing and harvesting medicinal plants to preparing tinctures, essential oils, and infusions. It also includes information on how to make your own natural antibiotics, which can be especially helpful in today's world, where antibiotic-resistant bacteria are becoming increasingly common.

PART 01

Chapter 01 Properties of medicinal plants

Medicinal plants are widely used in home, traditional, and alternative medicine. Medicinal plants contain active compounds that can affect the body. The properties of medicinal plants depend on various factors, including the type of plant, the parts used, and preparation methods. Some medicinal plants are effective at treating various ailments, while others are only useful for specific conditions.

Medicinal plants are used by cultures all over the world, both for their medicinal properties and for their nutritional value. The use of medicinal plants has been documented in China since ancient times, and many people living in developing countries still depend on them as the only form of healthcare they can afford.

Medicinal plants often prevent or treat many ailments, including heart disease, diabetes, cancer, etc.

Different plants have different effects on the human body. Some plants may be toxic if ingested in large amounts, so you must know which ones to use and avoid.

In addition to identifying different types of plants and their uses, it's also helpful to know how they can affect your health.

One of the most important things to remember about medicinal plants is that they're not composed of a single compound. Most plants have complex mixtures of chemicals, many of which have different effects on your body.

The active compounds in medicinal plants are often complex mixtures that work together to produce beneficial effects, not just one combination. For example:

- Aloe vera sap contains more than 200 different compounds (including vitamins A and C). It also contains various minerals such as calcium, magnesium, and potassium.
- Stinging nettles contain high levels of iron, vitamins A and C, and other nutrients like folate (folic acid), zinc, and selenium - all important for good health!

Not all medicinal plants are equally useful. Some have been tested in clinical trials and proven effective, while others have yet to be fully researched.

It's important to be aware of this fact when considering the use of any herbal medicine.

Herbal supplements are usually cheaper than conventional prescription medications with similar effects, but the FDA doesn't regulate them. This means you can only sometimes trust the label on an herbal supplement! The

FDA has rules about what information manufacturers must include on their labels and how it should be presented. It also has standards for testing products before they can be sold in stores or online.

The lack of regulation means that any claims made about herbal supplements may not be valid--and since many people take these products for medical reasons (like lowering cholesterol), they are at risk of being harmed by false advertising claims.

Traditional medicinal plants of India

The traditional medicinal plants of India are well known for their therapeutic properties and have been used by people for centuries.

The following table provides a list of some of the most popular ones:

- Awani (carom seeds) - is said to aid digestion, reduce flatulence and act as an expectorant. This spice has also been used as an insect repellent. It can be taken with water or honey as part of a daily routine for better health.

Medicinal plants of Indian origin

Indian medicinal plants are the most used in the world. They have been used since ancient times and continue to be used by many people worldwide today. The use of Indian medicines has been recorded from as early as 2000 B.C. and continues till date, with more than 80% of people using them regularly for health benefits.

Medicinal properties of medicinal plants

Medicinal plants have been used for centuries to treat a variety of ailments and diseases. These plants contain various chemical compounds that have medicinal properties, including anti-inflammatory, antibacterial, antifungal, and antiviral activity. Traditional medicines from medicinal plants have been used to treat conditions such as malaria, cancer, diabetes, and cardiovascular diseases. Additionally, medicinal plants have been used to relieve pain, reduce stress and anxiety, and improve overall health and well-being. Scientific research has confirmed the efficacy of many medicinal plants, and some of their compounds have been isolated and synthesized for use in modern medicine. The use of medicinal plants remains an important area of research, potentially providing new treatments for various diseases.

The medicinal properties of medicinal plants have been recognized for centuries and have been used in traditional medicine practices around the world. These plants contain various active compounds that have been shown to have therapeutic effects on the human body. The most commonly used medicinal plants include ginseng, echinacea, and chamomile. Ginseng, for example, has been found to boost energy levels, improve cognitive function, and enhance immune function. Echinacea is known for its ability to boost the immune system and reduce inflammation, while chamomile is often used as a natural remedy for insomnia and anxiety. As research continues to uncover the benefits of medicinal plants, they are increasingly being integrated into modern healthcare practices.

The Ayurvedic approach to plant-based medicine

The Ayurvedic approach to plant-based medicine is a holistic and natural method of healing the body, mind, and soul. Rooted in ancient Indian philosophy, Ayurveda emphasizes the importance of balancing the three doshas-Vita, Pitta, and Kaph- to promote optimal health. Herbs and plants play a crucial role in Ayurvedic medicine, as they are used to create powerful remedies tailored to individual needs. Ayurvedic practitioners believe plants contain an innate intelligence that can be harnessed through proper preparation and dosage. The use of plant-based medicine in Ayurveda offers a safe, effective, and sustainable approach to healthcare that aligns with the body's natural rhythms and promotes long-term wellness.

Herbal medicines are formulated based on the individual's body type and specific health needs. Ayurvedic practitioners believe that plants have unique healing properties that can be harnessed to treat a wide range of ailments. Unlike conventional medicine, Ayurveda considers the whole person, including their physical, emotional, and spiritual health, when determining the appropriate course of treatment. Individuals can holistically achieve optimal health and well-being by incorporating Ayurvedic principles into plant-based medicine.

Medicinal plants are the most commonly used remedy for many diseases.

Medicinal plants are the most commonly used remedy for many plants. Medicinal plants have many benefits, and they can be used as medicine to treat many diseases. Medicinal plants have been utilized for centuries as remedies for various diseases and illnesses. They are the most common source of medicine in many parts of the world, especially in developing countries where access to modern healthcare is limited. These plants are rich in therapeutic compounds that help prevent and treat a wide range of ailments. Medicinal plants have gained popularity in recent years, with an increasing number of people turning to natural remedies for their health needs. Scientific research has also shown that some medicinal plants have potent pharmacological properties, making them useful in developing new drugs. Overall, medicinal plants are a vital resource in the fight against diseases and can potentially improve global health.

They are usually found growing in areas where they can easily access sunlight and water.

When looking for medicinal plants, it is important to understand that they are usually found growing in areas where they can easily access sunlight and water. This means that if you want to grow your own medicinal plants, it is best to pick an area with plenty of light and moisture.

They may also grow on mountains or rocky cliffs, depending on their species.

Certain plant species have adapted to grow on mountains or rocky cliffs, where the environment may be harsh and challenging. These plants have developed unique adaptations, such as deep roots for stability and efficient water uptake or small, thick leaves to reduce water loss through transpiration. Depending on their species, these plants may thrive in high altitudes or arid conditions, where other plants may struggle to survive. They play an important role in maintaining the ecosystem, providing habitats and food sources for other organisms. The ability of these plants to grow in extreme environments highlights the resilience and adaptability of nature.

Certain species of plants have adapted to grow in difficult environments, such as mountainous regions and rocky cliffs. These plants have developed specialized traits to cope with these harsh conditions, such as the ability to anchor themselves firmly to rocky surfaces and withstand strong winds. The type of plant that can grow in these areas will vary depending on the specific species, as not all plants can thrive in such environments. Nevertheless, the ability of these plants to grow in challenging landscapes is a testament to their resilience and capacity to adapt to different conditions.

Medicinal plants' properties depend highly on the soil in which they grow.

- The chemical composition of herbs varies depending on their habitat and environment, which can affect their medicinal value.
- Medicinal plants' properties depend highly on the soil in which they grow. The quality of soil plays a crucial role in determining the potency of medicinal plants. The ground provides nutrients, water, and minerals that facilitate the growth of plants. Medicinal plants require specific conditions for optimal growth and development. The soil's pH level, moisture content, and nutrient composition affect the plant's biochemical makeup and the potency of the active compounds present in them. Understanding the soil requirements of medicinal plants is essential for their cultivation and harvesting. Proper soil management practices can enhance the therapeutic properties of the plants and ensure the production of high-quality medicinal products.

- The properties of medicinal plants have been studied for centuries, and their benefits are well documented. However, what is less well known is that the soil these plants grow is vital in determining their medicinal properties. The quality of the soil can influence the concentration of various nutrients and minerals in the plant, which can impact the plant's ability to produce certain chemicals and compounds that have medicinal properties. Additionally, the soil's pH level can also affect the availability of these nutrients and minerals to the plant. Therefore, it is important to recognize the significance of the soil in the cultivation and utilization of medicinal plants.

Many of these plants have been used by humans for centuries with no side effects or adverse reactions.

- The American Academy of Pediatrics recommends that parents avoid giving children under two any medication, including herbal remedies.
- Throughout history, humans have relied on plants for a myriad of purposes, including medicinal, nutritional, and cultural uses. Many of these plants have been used for centuries without reported side effects or adverse reactions. This is a testament to the efficacy and safety of these traditional remedies. While scientific research has validated the benefits of some of these plants, others remain unexplored. However, it is important to note that not all plants are safe for human consumption, and proper caution and consultation with a healthcare professional should always be exercised. Nonetheless, the long history of safe usage of many plants highlights the potential for natural remedies in improving human health and wellness.
- Human beings have utilized numerous plants for centuries without any negative consequences or unfavorable reactions. This is a testament to the natural healing properties that these plants possess. Many cultures worldwide have relied on traditional herbal medicine to treat various ailments, and the effectiveness of these remedies is well-documented. However, it is crucial to acknowledge that not all plants are safe for consumption or external use, and caution must be exercised when using any herbal remedy. It is always recommended to consult a healthcare professional before incorporating new herbal treatments into a wellness routine.

Medicinal plants can be broken down into two distinct types:

- Plants that have been used in traditional medicine for centuries, such as aloe vera, ginger, and ginkgo biloba. These herbs have a long history of use and are generally considered safe when taken in small amounts by adults. You can find these herbal remedies at most health food stores or online.
- Plants that are new to Western medicine but that have shown promise in scientific studies, such as ashwagandha (an Ayurvedic herb), turmeric, and green coffee bean extract. These herbs may be less well-

known than some of the traditional medicines listed above, but they're still worth exploring if you're looking for natural ways to treat a medical condition or improve your overall health.

Medicinal plants can affect the animal body in various ways, including both direct and indirect processes.

What exactly is a medicinal plant? A medicinal plant is any species of the Kingdom Plantae that has been used in the preparation of remedies for diseases, disorders, and other health problems. The use of plants as medicine has been documented throughout history. There are many reasons why medicinal plants have been used since ancient times: they have fewer side effects than synthetic drugs; they are often cheaper; they're readily available in nature; some are easy to grow at home or on your window sill; some have antibacterial properties that can help fight infections (e.g., ginger); others contain chemicals with strong anti-inflammatory properties (e.g., turmeric).

Medicinal plants have been used in traditional medicine for their purported health benefits for centuries.

These plants contain active compounds known to possess therapeutic properties that can help alleviate symptoms and promote healing. The use of medicinal plants has been documented in various cultures around the world, and many continue to be used today. While modern medicine has largely replaced traditional remedies, the importance of medicinal plants cannot be understated. Research has shown that many plants possess powerful medicinal properties that can potentially treat a wide range of health conditions. As such, the study of medicinal plants remains an important area of research in medicine.

Many of these medicinal plants are still widely used in modern medicine, with pharmaceutical companies incorporating their active ingredients into various drugs and supplements. However, it is important to approach the use of medicinal plants with caution, as some may have harmful side effects or interact with other medications. As such, seeking advice from a qualified healthcare professional before using any medicinal plant is crucial.

Medicinal plants can be classified into three groups: herbs ("herbal remedies"), spices, and aromatics. Herbs are generally grown as annuals or perennials in temperate climates. Still, they can also be grown as tender perennials in warmer climates, such as those found in Southern California or Florida.

Some medicinal plants are effective at treating a variety of ailments, while others are only useful for specific conditions. For example, lavender oil may be your best bet if you have headaches or muscle soreness. If you have allergies or anxiety issues, however, chamomile tea might be better suited to your needs.

When considering the benefits of using medicinal plants as part of your health regimen:

- Check with your physician before beginning any new treatment plan (and if anything, in particular, concerns them). Your doctor may also recommend taking supplements alongside herbal remedies, so make sure they're aware of all the steps being taken!

Many medicinal plants can be toxic if taken incorrectly.

For this reason, it is important to consult a trained herbalist before using any plant medicinally. It is important to recognize that while many medicinal plants can offer significant health benefits, they can pose a risk if not used correctly. Ingesting certain plants in incorrect doses or preparation methods can lead to toxicity and adverse effects. It is critical to consult with a trained healthcare professional or herbalist before incorporating any medicinal plants into one's health regimen. It is also essential to source plants from reputable suppliers and thoroughly research their potential side effects and interactions with other medications. Despite their potential risks, when used correctly, medicinal plants can offer a safe and natural alternative to traditional medications.

The most important thing to know about medicinal plants is that they can be very helpful. Still, talking with your doctor before taking any herbal supplement or alternative treatment is important, especially if you are taking other medications.

Medicinal plants have properties.

Some properties are useful in treating diseases, while others are not. For example, some medicinal plants may be painkillers or reduce fevers. Others can be used to treat infections or as an antidote for poisons that cause illness or death if left untreated.

Medicinal plants have been used since ancient times for their healing powers. Many people still rely on them today for their medical needs because they're easy to find and grow in almost any climate around the world (except Antarctica).

Medicinal plants have been used for thousands of years.

A study of plants in the Amazon rainforest has revealed that they contain more than 420 chemical compounds that may be useful as medicines. We are now beginning to understand how these compounds work together to produce their medical effects. Researchers are also studying how Western medicine can help heal tropical diseases. It is important to protect the rainforest because it is a source of many important medicinal plants.

Medicinal plants have been used for thousands of years.

The practice of using medicinal plants dates back to ancient civilizations. The first known written record of herbal medicine was found in the Ebbers Papyrus, which dates back to 1550 BCE and is thought to be the oldest medical document still in existence today.

The Chinese Pharmacopoeia (Ben Cao Gang Mu), written between c. 200 BCE-200 CE, was another early example of this knowledge being recorded and shared with others.

The rainforests of the Amazon Basin are home to over half of the world's plant species. They are also an important source of medicines that have been used for thousands of years by indigenous people in South America and Africa, who have developed a sophisticated understanding of how plants can be used as medicine.

Science has recently begun to catch up with this ancient knowledge. A study published in Science Advances last year showed that more than 420 different chemical compounds were present in 16 medicinal plants growing in Brazil's Para State--more than half had not previously been identified by Western science.

We are now beginning to understand how these compounds work together to produce their medical effects. For example, the active ingredients in cannabis have been shown to interact with receptors in our brains that control pain and mood. This discovery led scientists to develop medicines that target those same receptors with fewer side effects than traditional painkillers like morphine.

Now that we've got this basic understanding of medicinal plants' active ingredients let's look at some of the most promising herbal supplements on the market today!

Researchers are also studying how Western medicine can help heal tropical diseases. For example, University of Utah researchers have found that a chemical in licorice root may be able to kill the bacteria that causes typhoid fever and cholera.

Many civilizations have used medicinal plants, and they continue to provide important remedies for modern-day health problems.

For example, the Chinese have been using medicinal herbs for thousands of years. In fact, some of their medicines were taken from plants that grew in what is now North America!

The first recorded use of a medicinal plant dates back to 2700 BC.

The ancient Egyptians used an infusion from the flowering tops of marshmallows (Althea officinalis) as a demulcent and soothing agent for the eyes, mouth, throat, and lungs.

In China, the Huangdi Beijing ("Yellow Emperor's Inner Canon"), dating from the 3rd century BCE, lists herbs used for various ailments, including gingivitis. The ancient Greeks cultivated medicinal plants on an extensive scale.

Many plants were considered sacred and used only by shamans or religious leaders.

Medicinal plants were also common in ancient China, where they were believed to have a connection with the gods.

Ancient Egyptians used different herbs to treat various illnesses.

For example, they would grind up the leaves of a plant called feverfew and make them into tea for headaches or nausea. The ancient Greeks also relied on medicinal plants for their health needs--they even had doctors who specialized in herbal medicine!

Ancient Romans had many herbs and spices in their diet for taste and health benefits.

The Romans used a lot of herbs and spices in their diet, both for taste and health benefits.

The ancient Romans consumed foods rich in Vitamin K (such as leafy greens), which helps keep your heart healthy and strong. They also ate foods high in antioxidants like flavonoids, which help fight diseases like cancer and heart disease.

In India, Ayurvedic medicine was developed thousands of years ago and remains a popular form of treatment today. In China, acupuncture has been practiced since at least 2700 BCE; it's believed to have originated with the Yellow Emperor Huangdi Beijing.

The earliest records of Chinese herbalism date back to 2700 BC as well.

In fact, one of the earliest known medical texts was written by a Chinese emperor named Shen Nong and is called The Divine Husbandman's Classic of Materia Medica (whom we now call "the father of Chinese medicine").

The practice continued through ancient times until it spread westward during the Silk Road era, influencing Western herbalism and medicine.

Modern scientists are studying traditional techniques to gain insights into plant-based medicines.

Medicinal plants have been used for thousands of years. Modern scientists are studying traditional techniques to gain insights into plant-based medicines.

The use of medicinal plants dates back thousands of years when people would gather them in the wild or grow them on their farms and gardens. They believed these plants could heal wounds and cure illnesses, so they experimented with different methods of preparation: grinding leaves into powders, steeping roots in hot water, and boiling whole flowers in oil or butterfat (a process called enfleurage).

Herbal remedies have been used since ancient times.

The earliest record of herbal medicine dates back to around 2700 BCE, when Sumerians recorded the use of herbs for medicinal purposes in cuneiform tablets. Herbs were also used by the ancient Egyptians, Greeks, Romans, and other cultures throughout history.

Herbal remedies are sometimes used instead of prescription drugs.

Herbal remedies are often made from plant parts and other natural ingredients. These include leaves, roots, seeds, and bark. Herbal medicines can treat pain or other health problems such as coughs and colds.

Some herbs can be harmful if not properly used.

If you're thinking about using herbs for medicinal purposes, it's important to research them thoroughly. Some herbs can be harmful if not properly used. For example, ivy leaves are often used in teas to treat the common cold or flu but can cause skin irritation if you come into contact with them directly.

Herbs can also be helpful when combined with prescription medications.

Herbs are not drugs, and they do not have side effects. Herbs work best when used with other natural remedies, like acupuncture or massage therapy.

Many people use herbal medicines because they feel safer than pharmaceutical drugs, but some herbal products may not be safe or effective.

- Some herbs are not regulated by the U.S. Food and Drug Administration (FDA) and do not have to meet the same standards as prescription medications. As a result, these products may contain different amounts of active ingredients than what is listed on their labels and could be contaminated with other substances that could cause harm if taken in too high a dose or for an extended period of time.
- Some herbs can interact with other drugs you're taking--sometimes causing serious side effects.

Medicinal plants have been used for thousands of years. They've been used so long that they're part of our DNA. It's in our blood--literally! Our ancestors used these plants as medicine because they were effective, safe (and sometimes even delicious).

It wasn't until the 20th century that synthetic drugs came onto the scene, which means we only have about 100 years' worth of data on their effects compared to thousands of years' worth of medicinal herbs and spices.

Herbs have been used in traditional healing practices for thousands of years.

In fact, many herbs have been used for so long that we don't even know their exact origins. But it's safe to assume that herbal remedies were popularized by ancient civilizations before the advent of modern medicine.

Medicinal plants have been used for thousands of years. Some people believe that natural remedies are more effective than pharmaceuticals, but modern medicine has developed over time, with new treatments being developed daily.

One of the main reasons people turn to herbal remedies is because they are less invasive than Western medicine. For example, if you have a headache, you can take an aspirin or ibuprofen tablet to ease the pain and reduce inflammation. These medications stop the production of prostaglandins (a type of hormone) that causes inflammation.

In contrast, traditional Chinese medicine uses acupuncture needles to stimulate nerves and blood vessels under the skin's surface in order to relieve pain and reduce swelling around an injury site. Although both treatments involve inserting something into your body--one with pills or capsules, one with needles--acupuncture does not have any side effects like those caused by aspirin or ibuprofen because it doesn't directly interact with any organs in your body beyond stimulating nerves near where pain occurs (which may also help explain why some people prefer this treatment).

Herbal supplements can be found as dietary supplements or medications and may consist of one herb or many herbs combined in a single product. Herbal supplements often treat various health conditions, including pain, headaches, and insomnia.

In addition to their use in traditional medicine, some herbal products have been approved by the U.S. Food & Drug Administration (FDA). These include:

Herbs are believed to positively affect various conditions, from heart problems to depression. Still, research is limited due to funding constraints and lack of interest from pharmaceutical companies.

In addition to their medicinal properties, many herbs are edible and used in cooking.

Medicinal plants have been used for thousands of years.

The earliest known use of medicinal plants dates back to around 2700 BC, in ancient Egypt, where they were used as part of the embalming process.

Medicinal plants are any plant with a chemical compound that can treat or prevent disease in humans and animals. The chemical compounds found in these plants can be extracted and purified for use as medications or supplements.

Most medicinal plants are not harmful.

Many of them are used as food and medicine by people worldwide. The word "medicinal" means "having healing properties." Medicinal plants have been used for centuries to treat various ailments and illnesses.

Medicinal plants have been used for thousands of years to treat diseases and promote health. But some plants, like poppies and cannabis, also produce drugs that can be dangerous or addictive.

The use of medicinal plants is an important part of traditional medicine systems around the world. In Western countries, many different types of herbal medicines are available on prescription from a doctor or health professional (such as homeopathy). Herbal remedies may help you feel better if you have an illness or condition, but they won't cure it completely - they just relieve your symptoms. At the same time, you wait for your body's natural healing processes to work properly again.

The use of medicinal plants has declined in Western countries in recent decades but is still common in developing countries.

Medicinal plants have been used for thousands of years by many cultures around the world. These natural remedies have been used to treat everything from headaches to snake bites and even cancer.

Plants can help us feel better.

Many different types of plants have been used for thousands of years by people all over the world. Some plants are used to treat illness, others for their beauty and smell, and others provide food or clothing.

Medicinal plants have been used for thousands of years.

The earliest known use of medicinal plants dates back to the Stone Age when people used them to treat illnesses and injuries.

Medicinal plants have been used for thousands of years. The earliest known illustration of a medicinal plant is from an Egyptian papyrus dated 1550 BCE.

More than 80,000 plant species have been used for medicinal purposes.

A study published in Science Advances found that one-quarter of modern medicines can be traced back to traditional herbal remedies. These include treatments for malaria and tuberculosis, which both started out as plants.

Medicinal plants are often used as an alternative to synthetic drugs because they're less expensive and don't always have side effects like those associated with prescription medications.

More than half of the world's population uses herbal remedies as their first choice for healthcare.

Herbal remedies have been used for thousands of years. More than half of the world's population uses herbal remedies as their first choice for healthcare, and they are safe, effective, and affordable.

Herbal medicines are made from plants that grow naturally in different parts of the world. These natural medicines contain active ingredients called phytochemicals (Phyto means "plant"). Phytochemicals have been shown to have many health benefits, such as fighting cancer cells or boosting immunity by helping your body fight infections better than it can on its own.

There are many different types of medicinal plants, and they may be useful in treating a wide range of conditions. Some plants can treat skin infections, while others may help reduce inflammation or relieve pain.

Some herbs have have anti-cancer properties, including pomegranate seed oil (which has been shown to prevent the growth of breast cancer cells), green tea (which slows down tumor growth), and turmeric (a spice used in South Asian cooking).

Medicinal plants help us stay healthy.

Many plants around us have medicinal properties. In today's fast-paced world, medicinal plants have not been seen as a viable alternative to modern medicine. However, many scientific studies and research are being carried out to prove their benefits in keeping people healthy. There are many types of medicinal plants found all over the world, but the ones that have been used for centuries are particularly effective in maintaining proper balance in our body's systems. Herbal supplements have been shown to have fewer side effects than pharmaceutical drugs and offer great health benefits. Medicinal plants can aid in the treatment of illnesses and other health problems.

Many plants around us have medicinal properties.

You can find medicinal plants around you. There are many plants around us that have medicinal properties, but we don't know about them because we don't pay attention to them.

In today's fast-paced world, medicinal plants have not been seen as a viable alternative to modern medicine.

However, there are many reasons why it should be considered:

- The cost of these herbs is much lower than many prescription drugs and over-the-counter medications.
- Some plants have been used for centuries to treat specific ailments; therefore, we can trust that their efficacy has been proven over time by others who have used them before us.

In addition to being cost-effective and safe (when taken correctly), some herbs are also easy on our environment because they don't require pesticides or chemicals to grow well in your garden!

Scientists are studying the medicinal plants used for centuries to see if they can be used in modern medicine and healthcare.

Many types of medicinal plants are found worldwide, but the ones that have been used for centuries are particularly effective in maintaining proper balance in our body's systems.

Medicinal plants can be used to treat a wide range of illnesses and conditions. They can also help you feel better if you're feeling under the weather or just want some extra energy.

Herbal supplements have been shown to have fewer side effects than pharmaceutical drugs and offer great health benefits.

Many people know that herbs can be used as medicine but don't know how to take them. There are many ways to use herbal supplements: you can brew them into teas or infuse oils with them; you can even make tinctures out of them!

Medicinal plants can aid in the treatment of illnesses and other health problems

Medicinal plants have been used for thousands of years to treat many different conditions. These include:

- Pain relief
- Digestion support
- Anti-aging properties (that's right, you can slow down the aging process by using medicinal plants)

Herbs can help improve sleep and relieve stress.

- Chamomile: An herb that has been used for centuries to treat anxiety and insomnia, chamomile also helps with heart health, digestion, skin conditions, and even menstrual pain. It has a calming aroma when inhaled or ingested in tea form.
- Passionflower: This herb is often used to treat insomnia because it contains flavonoids that promote restful sleep by reducing anxiety levels before bedtime. Passionflower can also be used as an herbal remedy for headaches caused by stress or anxiety; one study found that taking passionflower extract during the day reduced depression among adults with chronic pain conditions such as fibromyalgia or arthritis.

Plants often treat skin conditions such as acne, eczema, and psoriasis.

Plants contain many organic compounds that have medicinal properties. Some plants' leaves are used to treat skin problems like acne and eczema.

Many herbs have antioxidant properties that help to fight free radicals.

- Antioxidants are natural compounds found in plants that can help prevent damage caused by free radicals.
- Free radicals damage cells and tissues, causing them to age prematurely.

Medicinal plants can be used to cure many illnesses. They have been used for generations and are still used today as a form of treatment.

Medicinal plants are more affordable than going to the clinic.

The cost of going to the clinic is very high. You have to pay for transportation, food, accommodation, and consultation fees, which can run into thousands of naira. Medicinal plants are cheaper because they are readily available at home or from your local market.

There are many kinds of medicinal plants; some help the heart and others for arthritis, for example.

The medicinal plants we use to help us remain healthy can be found in forests and mountains and on our own doorstep.

Medicinal plants have been used for centuries to cure illnesses. Many of the herbs we use today are still used to treat various ailments.

The World Health Organization (WHO) estimates there are at least 50,000 medicinal plants in use around the world today. The WHO also estimates that 80 percent of these are useful in treating some disease or condition.

Many of the plants used in medicine today are native to North and South America.

For example, the coca plant leaves have been chewed for thousands of years by people in Peru, Bolivia, and Colombia to combat fatigue and hunger. The active ingredient in tea leaves--caffeine--is also found in many other plants, including coffee beans and kola nuts.

The practice of plant-based healthcare is called ethnomedicine.

Ethnomedicine is the practice of plant-based healthcare. It's also known as ethnopharmacology, and it can be used to treat a variety of ailments, including:

- Pain

- Anxiety
- Infections, such as colds and flu
- Chronic conditions like diabetes or high blood pressure

European settlers first brought many medicinal plants to North America in the 16th century, such as tobacco and coca leaves. Native herbs used these plants for healing purposes long before Europeans arrived on their land. For example, they would chew on willow bark to relieve pain or boil roots from certain trees to make medicine.

Medicinal plants help us stay healthy.

Most of us don't think about the health benefits of plants until we're sick, but they can be an important part of a healthy lifestyle. If you want to get the most out of your food and keep yourself in good shape, try adding herbs and spices!

Some plants have medicinal properties and can be used for treatment of diseases.

Medicinal plants are used to cure various diseases. Some of these plants have been in use since ancient times and are still being used today. Some plants' medicinal properties can be used to treat diseases like diabetes, cancer, heart disease, etc.

It is important to know about the medicinal properties of plants so that you can use them in case of an emergency.

Elderberry: This is one of the most popular plants for treating colds, flu, cough, and sore throat. The berries contain antioxidants which help boost your immune system. You can eat elderberry jam or syrup made from them to treat these ailments.

- Medicinal plants are an important part of our history and should be a part of your future, too.
- There are many ways to use medicinal plants to help you stay healthy and prevent illness.

The medicinal properties of plants have been used for centuries to treat various diseases. Using herbs daily can help us maintain good health and lead happier lives.

Medicinal plants can improve physical or mental health

Medicinal plants are useful in treating various diseases, such as cancer or diabetes. In addition to curing disease symptoms, medicinal plants also prevent diseases by strengthening the immune system and improving physical fitness.

Medicinal plants are plants that can be used to prevent and treat illnesses. Some people believe medicinal plants effectively treat chronic conditions such as diabetes and high blood pressure. Others believe they can help with conditions that don't have a cure, like cancer.

Some examples of medicinal plants include:

- Aloe vera (Aloe barbadense) - this plant grows in warm climates and has been used since ancient times as a natural remedy for burns and skin irritations. It also helps relieve stomach pain caused by ulcers or irritable bowel syndrome (IBS).
- Ginseng (Panax ginseng) - this herb is native to China but now grows worldwide; it has been used since ancient times as medicine and food by many cultures worldwide. Some people believe it helps boost energy levels, while others say it fights off colds more effectively than over-the-counter medications do!

Medicinal plants can be found in your backyard

Some of the most effective medicinal plants are common weeds!

You might wonder how a weed could be good for you. Don't worry--weeds are very important to a healthy ecosystem. They help keep soil healthy and prevent erosion by holding down bare dirt with their extensive root systems (which can grow up to three feet deep). They also provide food and shelter for nearby animals; some even have medicinal properties!

Medicinal plants are used to treat various conditions, including pain and inflammation. The active ingredients in medicinal plants have been shown to have many therapeutic effects on the body.

These include:

- Antioxidant properties that help protect cells from damage caused by free radicals (molecules that can harm your DNA)
- Anti-inflammatory properties that reduce swelling and pain in your joints or muscles

Aloe vera

Aloe vera is a succulent plant found in the deserts of Africa, Asia, and America. It has been used for centuries to treat various ailments such as burns, wounds, and skin infections. The gel from its leaves is also used to treat other conditions, including arthritis, diabetes, and high cholesterol levels.

Amla

Amla is a medicinal plant that can be used to treat several health conditions. It has been used in Ayurvedic medicine for centuries to treat everything from fever and inflammation to asthma, constipation, heart disease, and diabetes. The main active ingredient in amla is vitamin C which helps prevent free radical damage to cells.

Ashwagandha

Ashwagandha is a medicinal plant used in Ayurvedic medicine for thousands of years. It's also known as Indian ginseng, which can grow in India, Sri Lanka, and Pakistan.

The name ashwagandha translates to "smell of horse" because the root smells like horse manure when dried out!

Arjuna

Arjuna is a woody plant that grows in tropical regions. It is also known as the Indian neem and belongs to the family Meliaceous. Arjuna's leaves, bark, and seeds have been used for medicinal purposes since ancient times.

Ayurveda (traditional Indian medicine) has been used as an astringent, anti-inflammatory agent, and tonic herb for its ability to purify the blood and remove toxins from the body.

Bael fruit

Bael is a tropical fruit that grows on a large tree in India, Bangladesh, Sri Lanka, and Indonesia. The bale tree can grow up to 30 meters tall and produce yellowish-green fruits with a hard outer skin containing one or two seeds. The pulp of the bale fruit has been used in Ayurvedic medicine since ancient times as it has many health benefits, including anti-inflammatory properties, antimicrobial activity against bacteria such as staphylococcus epidermidis (staph), salmonella typhi (salmonella) and Japanese encephalitis virus; antioxidant activity; antihypertensive effect on blood pressure; regulates blood glucose levels in diabetes mellitus type 2 patients; improves digestion by increasing secretion of digestive juices from stomach lining mucosa cells when taken before meals.

Belva

Belva is a medicinal plant that is used in Ayurvedic medicine. It belongs to the family Sapindaceous and is commonly known as bel or Bilwa in Hindi and Sanskrit, respectively. The plant has been used for centuries for its antioxidant, anti-inflammatory, and hepatoprotective properties and its ability to treat diabetes mellitus.

Brahmi

Brahmi is a flowering plant that has been used for thousands of years in Ayurveda, the traditional medicine system of India. Brahmi comes from the Sanskrit word "Brahma," which means "the creator."

Brahmi is believed to have many benefits due to its ability to improve memory and concentration and calm the mind. It's also used as an anti-inflammatory agent for treating arthritis and eczema.

Buti klapa

Buti klapa is a medicinal plant that can be found in India, Nepal, and Pakistan. It is a perennial shrub with small yellow flowers. It has been used traditionally to treat diarrhea, dyspepsia, and coughs. Buti klapa contains alkaloids such as butyl choline, which have been shown to have anti-inflammatory properties in laboratory studies on mice.

In one study involving human volunteers who were given doses of Buti klapa extract for two weeks, researchers found that these doses did not affect heart rate or blood pressure.

Cactus (elephant foot yam)

The cactus is a medicinal herb that can be used to treat diabetes, fever, and other ailments. It has been used traditionally to treat several conditions, including:

- Constipation
- Diarrhea
- Dysentery

Medicinal plants are an integral part of traditional medicine around the world. They have been used for thousands of years and continue to be effective today in many cases where conventional treatments have failed.

Chapter 02 Native Herbs and their Use of Herbs

Native herbs have been used herbs for thousands of years. The Cherokee people believe that using herbs is a gift from the Creator. The Blackfeet tribe regarded yarrow as sacred because they believed it had healing properties. Paiute Indians used mullein to treat burns. The Ojibwa people used cattail roots as a remedy for skin ulcers. Many tribes, including the Cheyenne, Comanche, and Pueblo, used tobacco or other herbs during ceremonies and rituals. Native herbs have been using herbs to heal themselves and others for thousands of years -- some of which we still use today!

Native herbs have been used herbs for thousands of years.

The use of herbs by Native herbs dates back thousands of years. Herbs have been used by many cultures for healing and treating illnesses, infections, and wounds. Native herbs used herbs in many different ways, including applying them directly to the skin, inhaling or smoking them, or eating them as food. In addition to using plants for medicinal purposes, some tribes also believed that their use came from the Great Spirit or First People, who taught them how to cultivate these plants and how they could help improve health conditions such as infections. Many Native tribes have their unique names for certain herbs and plants that grow in their area. Still, there are some common ones as well, such as corn (Mayans), potatoes (Incan), pumpkins (Pueblo), strawberries (Cherokee), sunflowers (Sioux) cranberries (Massachusetts). Also, read on:

Native herbs have been used herbs for thousands of years.

Herbs are grown or gathered plants, dried out, and used in cooking or medicine. The leaves stems, and roots of herbs have different uses depending on their purpose. For example:

- Eating an herb like rosemary (the leaves) can help improve your memory by making it easier for oxygen to get into your brain cells.
- Sage (the leaves) has been shown to reduce inflammation caused by arthritis or psoriasis when taken internally; however, if applied directly onto the skin, it may irritate sensitive skin types, so be careful when applying this method!

Herbs were essential in Native life.

They were used for healing, cooking, and even spiritual rituals. Many herbs grew wild and were easily collected by Native herbs, who used them to make teas or medicines. Indigenous people have used herbs worldwide for thousands of years; some cultures still rely on them today.

The Native herbs used herbal remedies for everything from veterinary remedies to food preservation. They used herbs in their daily lives and during ceremonies, rituals, and traditional dances.

Herbs were also used by many tribes as part of religious ceremonies because they believed that the spirits of their ancestors resided in the plant's leaves or roots.

Herbs were also used in spiritual ceremonies and rituals.

Many Native tribes believe that herbs have healing powers and use them to treat illnesses and injuries. The Cherokee people believe certain herbs can be used as charms to protect against bad luck, improve their hunting skills, or help them find lost objects (see the Resources section).

The Native herbs had many uses for herbs. Some were used as medicine, others to make teas and infusions that could be drunk or smoked.

- Some herbs were considered sacred and could only be used by a medicine man or shaman.
- Other plants were used in ceremonies to cleanse the spirit and bring about visions.

Many Native cultures used plants and herbs to treat health conditions.

For example, the Cherokee people believed that a black cohosh plant could help ease menstrual cramps.

Many Native herbs also used herbal remedies for their spiritual practices. For example, the Ojibwe tribe would burn sage during a ritual cleansing ceremony before entering a sweat lodge or sacred space.

Some herbs were used for healing cuts, bites, and stings.

- The Cherokee used a plant called "fern" (also known as "bristly pussytoes") to help heal wounds. They would chew the leaves of this plant and then apply them to the wound. This helped stop bleeding and speed up healing by drawing out infection inside the body.
- Another herb that Native herbs used was called "black sage." It had antibacterial properties that helped heal infected wounds quickly by fighting off bacteria like staphylococcus aureus or MRSA (methicillin-resistant Staphylococcus aureus).

Other herbs were used for pain relief.

The Native herbs used cattails with a thick root that could be ground into a powder sprinkled on wounds to stop bleeding and help them heal faster. They also used willow bark, which contains an ingredient called silicon that made it similar to aspirin today.

The Native herbs also knew about plants that could simultaneously be used as medicine and food. One example is corn: they ate it but also ground up the kernels into flour and then baked them into bread or cakes (or even pancakes!).

Native herbs also smoked or chewed certain herbs as a form of treatment.

In addition to using herbs in cooking, Native herbs are also smoked or chewed certain herbs as a form of treatment. For example, they would smoke tobacco leaves to relieve pain and reduce fever. They chewed willow bark to ease headaches or treat sore muscles and used sagebrush to help with stomach aches.

The Native herbs also used herbs as a food source to improve their overall health. The leaves of the sweet wormwood plant were used to make tea, while the rootstock was boiled into a broth. The Iroquois tribe made tea from wild ginger roots that they drank when they had stomach pains or colds.

An example is using juniper berries in soups, breads, and other foods.

The use of herbs in Native food is a testament to their importance in wellness. For example, juniper berries have been used centuries as a spice and flavoring agent in soups, bread, and other foods. The berries contain essential oils that are believed to improve digestion by stimulating bile production in the liver.

Native herbs have been using natural medicines for thousands of years

The Native culture is rich in traditions and customs, which have helped them preserve their heritage as a people over thousands of years. One such example is the use of herbs to heal the body, mind, and spirit.

Native herbs have been used for thousands of years. The use of Native herbs is thought to date back as far as 10,000 years ago. These herbs are still used today by many people who believe that they can improve their health or provide other benefits.

Native herbs have been used herbs for thousands of years. The use of herbs by Native tribes was passed down orally from generation to generation.

Native herbs are used to treat various ailments, including infections, injuries, and respiratory problems.

They believed that plants had spirits or energies that could be harnessed by those who knew how to use them properly. In addition to using the plants themselves as medicine, many Native tribes also made teas out of certain herbs and drank them for their healing properties.

Native herbs were the first people to use herbs for healing. They also used them for religious ceremonies, rituals, and food.

Herbs such as sage and cedar were used for their medicinal properties and are still used today by Native herbs.

The Native herbs were also the first to cultivate corn, potatoes, and pumpkins. They used these plants as food sources and medicine. For example:

- The Incan people grew corn in South America. The Incans used it as a staple food; they also made flour from the kernels and drank chicha (a fermented beverage) from them (1).

- The Pueblo tribes grew pumpkins in what is now known as New Mexico and Arizona (2). They ate the fleshy fruit raw or roasted it over an open fire; they also dried strips of pumpkin leaves for tea or ground them into flour for baking bread like piki bread made from blue cornmeal flour mixed with water and then baked on hot stones set inside an earth oven lined with clay bricks called adobe ovens which gets its name from adobes--which means "adobe brick"--the Spanish word used by early settlers when building homes made out of mud bricks baked over fires

There are many similarities between Native medicine and modern medicine today.

For example, both use herbs to help with their healing practices. Native herbs would use plants that grew in the area they lived in, as well as ones that had been passed down from generation to generation. They also used herbs for ceremonial purposes, such as honoring their ancestors or asking for blessings from nature spirits. Similarly, modern medicine uses plants to treat illnesses but often does so in conjunction with other treatments like surgery or radiation therapy.

Both types of healing have been used successfully for thousands of years; however, there are differences between the two models that make each one unique:

- While some people may view Native herbs' methods as primitive because they didn't understand how certain things worked (like bacteria), this isn't necessarily true--they simply had a different approach based on what was available at the time (i.e., no microscopes).

Certain herbs were used for healing, others for protection, and others for ceremony.

Some of these herbs were used by all tribes, and some had specific uses that only certain tribes knew about.

Some examples of herbs that had multiple uses are:

- cedar - used as an incense during ceremonies as well as a medicine for coughs and colds; also used to make baskets and canoes

- black sage - burned as incense during ceremonies or rubbed on the skin during sweat baths (a type of sauna)

The Cherokee people were called the "Herbalists of the South" by early Europeans because they understood the importance of herbs. They used them for healing, food, and medicine. The Cherokee grew and harvested hundreds of plants that grew wild in their region, including mints, barks, leaves, and berries.

The Iroquois people believed in the concept of balance or harmony. Plants were believed to have a purpose, and if they were harvested too often, they would disappear.

Thus, Native herbs used herbs sparingly and respectfully.

In the past, Native herbs believed that their medicinal practices came from the First People or Great Spirit. They thought that these herbs were given to them by nature and had special powers.

Some people think of Native herbs as "savages" who lived in caves and ate wild plants for food. However, this is not true at all! In fact, some tribes lived in houses made out of wood or stone (like our houses today). And unlike Europeans at that time, who ate mostly meat and bread made with flour ground from wheat grain and yeast as an ingredient (bread), many tribes ate cornmeal mush made from dried kernels of corn mixed with water or milk instead--and sometimes beans!

Native herbs have always valued plants and their uses.

They are a part of the natural world, which was seen as sacred by many tribes. Native medicine is based on the belief that illness comes from natural causes and can be treated with natural remedies. They also believed that plants have spirits that can be used to heal people or animals if they are asked politely before taking them.

Native herbs have cultivated herbs from the earliest days of their civilization.

Herbs have been a part of Native culture for thousands of years. The first Native herbs were hunter-gatherers, but they soon began cultivating herbs as well. They discovered that some plants could be used to create medicine and help their people survive in the harsh environment.

Native herbs used herbal remedies for a wide variety of ailments.

- For example, they would brew tea from the leaves of willow trees to reduce fevers or apply salves made from yarrow or calendula flowers to treat wounds. These natural treatments were often more effective than European medicines and had fewer side effects.

Plants were used as medicine, food, clothes, and decorations.

They used them to heal wounds and sicknesses and to make their homes more comfortable. Some plants were also used as clothing or blankets to keep them warm in the harsh climate of North America.

Some plants can be used for more than one purpose.

For instance, the wood of the American chestnut can be used to make furniture, while its leaves have been used as a food source by Native herbs.

- Medicinal plants are often easily recognizable by their flowers, fruit, or leaves.
- Some plants have been used for centuries by Native herbs to treat illnesses and injuries.

The bark of trees was often used in healing poultices.

Native herbs are also used herbs to treat wounds, such as by applying them directly to the skin or using them to create a poultice. They would crush up leaves and stems or boil them down into tea. The leaves from various plants were often used for this purpose as well, such as lemon balm (Melissa officinalis), which is still grown today for its medicinal properties and ability to soothe digestive problems like heartburn.

Roots were also used to make healing poultices.

A poultice is a soft mass of herbs applied directly to the skin, soaking up moisture and releasing its active ingredients into the body. Native herbs used a variety of roots for this purpose, including bearberry (Arctostaphylos uva-ursin), plantain (Plantago major), and Solomon's seal.

Herbs are found in many different places, including forests, streams, and mountains. The most common herbs are sage, thyme, mint, and rosemary.

Native herbs have been used herbs for thousands of years. Herbs were an important part of Native life, and they still are today. Many people use herbs to treat illnesses or improve their health.

Native herbs have been used herbs for thousands of years. The use of Native herbs is thought to date back as far as 10,000 years ago. The use of herbs by Native tribes was passed down orally from generation to generation.

The natives of North America were among the first people to develop an extensive knowledge of medicinal plants and their properties. Their use of these herbs and plants was a key component in their survival as they learned how to care for themselves, their families, and their communities through herbal remedies that could be easily grown or gathered in the wild.

The Cherokee people believe that the use of herbs is a gift from the Creator.

They say there are two kinds of medicine: herbal and spiritual. Anyone can learn the former, while the latter comes only through dreams and visions.

The Cherokee have been using natural remedies for thousands of years but didn't always know what they were doing! Their main goal was to heal their patients as quickly as possible so they could return them to their duties in life--or even save their lives when necessary.

The Blackfeet tribe regarded yarrow as sacred because they believed it had healing properties.

Native herbs use this herb to treat wounds, reduce pain, and promote healing. The Blackfeet also applied yarrow to the skin to help heal cuts and scratches.

Yarrow can be found growing in many places throughout North America. It grows wild in meadows and fields all over North America; however, it can also be cultivated easily at home if you're interested in growing your own herbs!

Paiute Indians used mullein to treat burns.

The leaves of this herb are poulticed over a burn and then wrapped in a cloth bandage, which may be soaked in water before application. They believed that mullein had healing properties because it was one of the first plants to grow after fires had destroyed their land.

The Paiute weren't alone in their beliefs about mullein; other Native tribes also used it for medicinal purposes, including treating colds and coughs by steeping the roots in hot water as well as soothing sore throats by gargling with an infusion made from dried leaves (which can also be smoked).

The Ojibwa people used cattail roots as a remedy for skin ulcers.

They also used the leaves to make a tea given to babies having trouble nursing. The tea was thought to help aid digestion and calm them down, so it was often given before bedtime.

Many tribes, including the Cheyenne, Comanche, and Pueblo, used tobacco or other herbs during ceremonies and rituals. The Cherokee tribe used sage in traditional Native ceremonies.

Native herbs have been using herbs to heal themselves and others for thousands of years -- some of which we still use today!

- The Native herbs used plants and herbs in almost every aspect of their lives, from medicine to food. They also used them to communicate with each other through rituals and ceremonies.
- Many tribes had their own doctors or healers who knew how to make all kinds of medicines from plants that grew around them. These doctors were called "medicine men" or "shamans."
- Native herbs used herbs to treat all kinds of ailments.

- They also used them for their medicinal properties, such as soothing skin irritations and easing pain.

Native herbs had a place in their lives for herbs.

They used them to treat illness, maintain health and generally improve quality of life.

They gathered plants from the wild and cultivated them on their land. They also traded with other tribes for plants that grew only in certain regions.

Many herbs had spiritual significance in addition to their medicinal uses.

For example, the root of the American orchid (Plantae: Orchidaceous) was used by Native tribes to treat snakebites and wounds. The plant is also believed to have supernatural powers and was used as a charm against evil spirits; it was often worn around the neck or placed in pouches on clothing.

Some Native herbs had a strong connection to the land and its herbs.

They used them as medicine and for other purposes, such as dyeing fabrics.

Many tribes in North America were known for their use of herbal remedies, which were passed down from generation to generation.

Some herbs were used as food as well as medicine.

Native herbs ate many different kinds of wild plants, such as the sweet potato and squash. They also grew crops such as corn, beans, and squash together in gardens called "Three Sisters." The Iroquois people made bread from pumpkins or squash seeds baked in hot ashes.

- Many Native tribes used herbs for healing.
- Some Native herbs also used plants to create dyes and medicines, such as the Cherokee, who used roots of the black cohosh plant to make a tea that could be used on cuts and bruises.
- The Cherokee used blue cohosh, a plant that can help with childbirth.
- The Native herbs used this herb to help women who were having trouble getting pregnant or had problems during pregnancy.
- The Navajo made a kind of tea from prickly pear cactus to help with diabetes.
- The Hopi have used juniper berries for hundreds of years as a remedy for colds, coughs, and sore throats.

The Apache cooked mullein root into soup to help with respiratory problems.

The Cherokee would chew the root of a plant called mountain balm and then spit it out over the sick person's body. They believed this would heal them.

Native herbs used many different herbs for healing purposes. Some of these herbs were used to treat illnesses, while others were used as food or spices.

Herbs were used for healing, love, and protection. For example, the Cherokee used black cohosh to treat menstrual cramps and liver problems. They also used it as an aphrodisiac to increase sexual desire in both men and women.

In addition to using herbs for medicinal purposes, they also used them in their spiritual ceremonies such as sweat lodges or vision quests where they would smoke tobacco leaves over hot coals before entering into a trance state induced by inhaling the fumes from burning sagebrush or sweetgrass incense sticks that were placed on top of large rocks heated in fire pits dug into the ground outside each lodge's entranceway.

- The Native herbs were the first to use plants to heal their sick.
- They recognized the healing qualities of many plants and learned how to use them effectively.
- Asthma
- Blood pressure issues
- Cancer treatment side effects (e.g., nausea)

Medicine men, or medicine women, as they are called today, have been a part of the American Indian culture for thousands of years. They have used herbs and other plants to heal their people.

The use of herbs by Native herbs dates back thousands of years. The earliest known human inhabitants of the Americas were hunter-gatherers who followed a nomadic lifestyle and used what they could find in their environment to supplement their diet and provide medicine. They relied on wild plants as food sources, medicinal remedies, and materials for clothing and shelter.

Tobacco was first cultivated by Native herbs who lived along the Mississippi River around 4500 BC; it was later introduced to Europeans during Columbus' voyages in 1492 CE (Common Era).

Early Native herbs used local plants to treat a variety of ailments, including stomach aches, fevers, and headaches. For example:

- The Navajo people crushed the leaves of sumac berries (Rhus trilobate) and mixed them with water to make a tea used for colds and coughs.
- The Zuni people chewed on the root of wild licorice (Glycyrrhiza alepidote) when they had sore throats or hoarseness from too much smoking or drinking alcohol; they also drank an infusion made from the roots as part of their tradition's puberty ceremony for young boys.

Native herbs sometimes combine herbs with traditional Chinese herbal medicine practices.

For example, they would use the herbs sassafras and sweet flag to treat colds and flu. These two plants have been shown to have antiviral properties in animal studies.

Many of these ancient herbal remedies are still used today.

One example is the use of ginseng to help people with diabetes who need to control their blood sugar levels. Another example is the use of goldenseal for colds, coughs, and sore throats.

Native herbs are experts in making use of herbs, plants, and trees found in the wilderness. This is because they have to survive on their own.

As they had no doctors or hospitals around them, they had to rely on nature's bounty to heal themselves from common ailments such as colds and fevers. They also used these natural remedies for treating more serious diseases like cancer, diabetes, and heart disease.

Early settlers learned that Native herbs used almost any plant they could find as medicine.

Native herbs used almost any plant they could find as medicine. Some of these plants were native to the Americas, but many came from other parts of the world. Europeans learned that Native herbs had been using herbs for centuries when they first arrived in North America. Many early settlers learned how to use herbs as medicines from Native tribes, including John Smith, who learned about herbs while living with the Powhatan tribe in Virginia.

Herbs were often used in teas, but sometimes they were smoked or chewed.

- The Tlingit tribe of the Pacific Northwest used a type of mint to treat stomach pain, colds, and headaches. They also used it as an insect repellent and rubbed it on their skin to keep mosquitoes away while they worked outside.
- The Cherokee used mullein leaves (a type of flower) as a remedy for sore throats and coughs when mixed with other herbs like gingerroot or lemon balm. Mullein flowers can be dried and stored for later use; once dried, they look like small brown balls packed with tiny seeds!

Native herbs would choose an herb based on what was needed.

The herbs had different properties, and each one had different uses. For example, if you were sick with a fever, you would drink some willow bark tea or boil the leaves of elderberry in water to make tea for yourself.

The first Americans were in the New World for over 15,000 years before the Europeans arrived. They had plenty of time to develop their own unique culture, and they used plants to help them with everything from food to medicine. The Native herbs used herbs like sagebrush or tobacco as everyday items like we might use a tissue or pen today--not just because they liked how it smelled but because these plants had practical uses as well!

The Native herbs used plants from the land all around them.

They also learned how to use other parts of an animal, such as its bones and skin. The Native herbs did not always grow crops; instead, they ate what was naturally available in their area during certain times of the year.

Medicine was often a mixture of several herbs, berries, or roots.

These would be boiled in water and then drunk as tea or applied to the skin as an ointment. Native herbs also used plants that were poisonous if eaten but which had medicinal properties when properly prepared.

Herbs were also used to treat common ailments such as colds and flu.

One of the most common ailments that Native herbs treated with herbal remedies was cold and flu. They used herbs like sassafras, ginger, and boneset to help their bodies fight off infection.

- Another common ailment was stomachache or indigestion, which could be caused by eating too much food or eating something that didn't agree with you. Here again, there were many different kinds of herbs they could use depending on what they thought might be causing it--and some were pretty funny! One example is using a mixture of peppermint leaves with water as an antacid.
- They were able to use plants for healing, food, clothing, and shelter. They also used plants to make tools such as bows and arrows.
- The Native herbs knew how to use plants in many ways: they made teas from leaves; they crushed roots into powder which they could then mix with water or fat (like bear grease) to create poultices; they boiled stems to make syrups; they even ate whole berries raw!
- They used them for medicine, food, clothing, and shelter.
- The Native herbs believed that all living things were connected by the Creator (God). They believed that all of nature was sacred and should be respected as part of the Creator's plan for us all.

The plants they used ranged from common weeds to rare herbs

For example:

- Wild turnip (aka prairie turnip) was boiled or roasted like potatoes and eaten as a vegetable by some tribes. It also had medicinal uses, such as relieving pain in the stomach when eaten raw. Some Native herbs would chew on the leaves of this plant if they had toothaches or sore gums.

Plants were used for medical purposes, food, alcohol, and clothing.

The Native herbs had many uses for plants. The Indians used plants as medicine or food. They also used them to make clothes, and they made alcohol out of some plants as well.

Native herbs didn't have hospitals. They treated and cured illnesses at home.

The Native herbs had to be very careful about what they ate because their food could be contaminated with bacteria or viruses that could make them sick. They knew which plants were safe to eat, so they wouldn't get sick from eating bad food.

Many herbs were used by tribes in the same way as modern doctors prescribe pharmaceuticals. For example, the Cherokee used dogwood berries to treat coughs and colds, while the Lakota Sioux used wild onion bulbs for stomach pain. The Cheyenne tribe would use buffalo berries as an antiseptic on wounds, while other Native herbs used cedar tree sap as an antiseptic against infections.

Some herbs were also used as recreational drugs or hallucinogens. The Chippewa tribe would make tea from wild ginger root, which they drank before going hunting because it made them more alert and focused on their prey; however, this same herb could cause hallucinations if taken in excess!

Tobacco was used by Native herbs for medicinal purposes, as well as for peace-making ceremonies. Some tribes used tobacco as a painkiller and to treat wounds.

Tobacco smoke was also used to cleanse the air in a lodge before guests arrived and during rituals or ceremonies.

Native herbs had an extensive knowledge of herbs and the ways in which they could be used. For example, the Cherokee made tea from the roots of black cohosh that was used as a blood tonic to help with menstrual cramps. They also used this herb to treat stomachaches and headaches.

The Native herbs also knew how to use herbs for medicinal purposes, such as treating wounds or infections with plants like bayberry bark or southernwood leaves.

The Native herbs used herbs for a variety of purposes, including medicinal.

The Native herbs were very good at using the resources that were available to them in their environment. They would use plants that grew in their area as medicine or food and also used the animals around them to help with hunting and trapping. The Native Indians had many uses for each plant they found in their natural habitat.

Many of the Native herbs have applications in natural healing today.

- Sage: Sage has been used by Native herbs for centuries as an herbal remedy for many ailments. It is believed that sage helps to ease pain and inflammation, control blood sugar levels, reduce cholesterol, and improve digestion.

- Ginseng (American): While several varieties of this herb are available today (like Korean or Chinese), American ginseng is considered superior because it grows wild in North America rather than Asia--and thus doesn't require replanting after harvesting like other types do. In addition to being an antioxidant-rich supplement that boosts energy levels naturally without caffeine or sugar overloads, research suggests it may also help fight off viruses such as colds or flu by boosting your immune system overall; keep in mind, though, that further studies are needed before any definitive conclusions can be made about their effectiveness against these types of illnesses!

Many of their healing methods were passed down orally, so we don't have many written records.

One example is the use of willow bark to treat pain, which was first recorded by a European doctor in 1633 but may have been used for centuries before then.

The first inhabitants of the Americas were Native herbs, who lived here for thousands of years. The earliest known evidence of humans in North America dates back to about 13,000 BC. When Europeans arrived in North America, there were over 500 different tribes living throughout what is now Canada and the United States.

The vast majority of these groups relied heavily on herbal remedies for treating ailments such as colds and fevers; however, they also used herbs for contraception as well as abortion practices (which were illegal during this time period).

We know that they used plants for healing and food.

The first Europeans to arrive in North America noticed the extensive use of herbs by Native herbs. The explorer Christopher Columbus observed that the Taino people of Hispaniola (now Haiti) used herbs in their healing practices. Later explorers described how other tribes also used herbs in their everyday life.

They used herbs to make medicines, both internally and externally.

The Native herbs were known to have used herbs for medicinal purposes as well as for making dyes and tannins. They also chewed on certain plants to keep their mouths fresh when they had nothing else to chew.

In addition to using plants for food, the Native herbs also made medicines from them. Many people today still use herbal remedies because they are cheaper than prescription drugs and work just as well (if not better).

Many Native tribes used different herbs in different ways.

Some tribes used herbs to heal, while others used them for spiritual purposes or as food.

For example, some tribes made tea from sage or mint leaves to clear their throats and lungs when they had a cold or cough. Other tribes would use cedar bark to make teas that helped ease pain from toothaches or headaches.

As you can imagine, there are many different plants that Native herbs would use for different ailments. Some tribes would rub their bodies with the leaves of certain plants to cure certain ailments.

Native herbs used herbs for many different purposes. To them, herbs were important because they provided food, medicines, and other things that made life easier.

The Native herbs used herbs for many different reasons. Some of them would use the leaves from trees for medicine, and others would use roots or flowers to make their clothes smell better or taste better when cooking dinner!

The Native herbs were known for their use of herbs. They used them as food and medicine, as well as in ceremonies and rituals. The Cherokee people believe that herbs are a gift from the Creator, who gave them this knowledge so they could heal themselves and others.

Chapter 03 Most Important Herbs

Herbs are a great way to add flavor and health benefits to your food. You should start if you're not using herbs yet in your cooking! Here are some of the most common herbs used in cooking.

Basil

Basil is a flowering plant in the mint family Liliaceae, native to tropical regions throughout the world. It is a bushy, woody shrub with green leaves and purple flowers that grows up to 2 feet tall. The most common variety of basil is sweet basil (Osmium Basilica), but there are many other varieties as well. Basil has been used for centuries as food and medicine by people worldwide; today, it's cultivated worldwide as an herb or spice for its distinct flavor and aroma.

Thyme

Thyme is a perennial herb that grows in most parts of the world. It can be used in cooking, cosmetics, and medicine. The leaves and flowers have been traditionally used to treat respiratory tract infections such as coughs, colds, and flu. They have also been used to help indigestion and asthma symptoms.

Sage

Sage is a perennial herb that grows in many parts of the world. The leaves are used for flavoring sausage, stuffing, and poultry dishes. Sage can be grown in containers on a patio or deck, but it prefers full sun and well-drained soil with a pH between 6 and 7 (slightly acidic).

Sage plants grow up to 2 feet tall with grayish-green leaves that have an earthy aroma when rubbed between your fingers. The flowers are small purple clusters borne on spikes at the ends of branches which bloom from July through September in most areas where it's grown--and sometimes through October if you live farther south than Zone 5!

Rosemary

Rosemary is a perennial herb that has a pine needle smell. It can be used in cooking, cosmetics, and herbal medicine. Rosemary has many uses in aromatherapy as well.

Oregano

Oregano is a member of the mint family and one of the most popular culinary herbs. It can grow up to 3 feet high, with purple flowers that bloom from July through September. Oregano is native to Europe, North America, and Asia but has also spread throughout much of the world.

Oregano has been used for centuries as both food and medicine by various cultures around the globe.

Parsley

Parsley is a leafy green herb that can be used in cooking but also has many medicinal uses.

- It cures kidney stones: Parsley contains high vitamin C levels, making it an effective remedy for kidney stones. The vitamin helps dissolve calcium oxalate crystals that form in the kidneys and cause pain during urination or blood in the urine.
- Good for digestion: Parsley contains fiber, antioxidants, and other nutrients that make it good for digestion. A study published by the American Journal of Clinical Nutrition found that drinking two cups (about 60 grams) of parsley tea daily helped reduce flatulence in people suffering from irritable bowel syndrome (IBS). Other studies have shown similar results with other types of teas made from different herbs, such as sage or rosemary.

Cilantro

Cilantro is a leafy herb that's used in many cuisines around the world. It's also known as coriander, which means "to sharpen" in Latin. The leaves and stems are used in cooking, while their roots are ground into powder and used to flavor foods like soups or stews.

Cilantro has been shown to have anti-inflammatory properties, which may help lower blood pressure by reducing inflammation throughout your body. Iron deficiency anemia affects about 1 billion people worldwide; cilantro contains more iron than spinach does, so eating this herb can help boost your intake of this essential mineral! Calcium helps strengthen bones; eating cilantro can help you meet your daily calcium needs without having to take supplements if you're not getting enough from your diet alone.

Mint

Mint is an herb used to flavor food and drinks. The leaves of mint are used in teas, jellies, and syrups and as a flavoring in candies and chewing gum.

Chamomile

Chamomile is a flower that can be used to make tea. It's also used in alternative medicine to treat anxiety, insomnia, and stomach issues. In addition to its medicinal properties, chamomile has been shown to have anti-inflammatory effects on the skin when applied topically.

Lavender

Lavender is a flowering plant in the mint family. It's native to the Mediterranean region, but it's now cultivated around the world for its fragrant flowers and essential oil. For centuries, lavender has been used as a medicinal herb to treat anxiety, stress, and insomnia.

Dandelion

Dandelion is a common weed that grows in your yard and on the side of the road. It's also used as an herbal medicine for treating kidney and liver problems. Dandelion has been used to treat gallstones, diabetes, urinary tract infections (UTIs), gout, and high cholesterol.

Dandelion leaves are more bitter than their roots or flower buds, but they're still edible raw or cooked in salads or soups. The root has a milder flavor than its leaves and can be eaten raw or cooked like potatoes -- try roasting them with olive oil until crispy on top!

Elderberry

Elderberry is a plant that grows in the wild. It has many medicinal properties and is used to treat colds, flu, and allergies, and is a tonic for the digestive system. The leaves can also be used to make an infusion (tea).

Elderberry tea has been shown to reduce fever in children suffering from acute respiratory tract infections (like colds or influenza). Elderberry syrup has proven effective against bacterial infections such as strep throat or tonsillitis when taken alongside antibiotics. Elderberry can also help with diarrhea by reducing inflammation of the intestines while speeding up the recovery time from stomach bugs like food poisoning or food allergies.

Ginger

Ginger is a rhizome that can be used to treat digestive problems, relieve nausea, and treat sore throats and colds. It's also known to be helpful in relieving arthritis pain due to its anti-inflammatory properties.

Turmeric

Turmeric is an herb that has been used in Ayurveda medicine for its anti-inflammatory properties. It's also a powerful antioxidant and has been shown to help with a variety of health conditions, including:

- Alzheimer's disease
- Cancer prevention and treatment (including breast cancer)
- Diabetes prevention and treatment (in people who are at risk for type 2 diabetes)

Lemon Balm

Lemon balm is a perennial herb with a lemon scent. It's used to make tea and can also be used as a medicinal herb. Lemon balm helps people sleep, soothe anxiety and stress, improve digestion, boost energy levels, and reduce depression symptoms.

Marshmallow Root

Marshmallow root is a great herb for the digestive system. It can help with constipation, diarrhea, and other G.I. issues.

Marshmallow root is also used as an anti-inflammatory agent to treat skin conditions such as eczema and psoriasis.

Valerian Root

Valerian root is a perennial, flowering herb that has been used since ancient times as a sedative. It's often used to treat insomnia and anxiety disorders like generalized anxiety disorder (GAD), post-traumatic stress disorder (PTSD), panic disorder and phobias.

Valerian also helps relieve depression symptoms such as irritability, fatigue, and restlessness by increasing levels of serotonin in the brain. This natural remedy can be used safely for up to six months at a time without experiencing any side effects or addiction risks; however, it should only be taken under supervision from your doctor if you're pregnant or breastfeeding because it could have some effect on your baby's health if taken regularly during pregnancy or lactation period.

Licorice Root

Licorice root is a plant that has been used for centuries to treat coughs, sore throats, and digestive problems such as heartburn and indigestion. It also treats ulcers, liver disease, and high blood pressure (hypertension).

Licorice root has been shown to lower cholesterol levels in the body by reducing the production of bile acids by the gallbladder; this may help prevent gallstones from forming in some people who already have them. Licorice can also reduce inflammation in the body by inhibiting an enzyme called cyclooxygenase-2 (COX-2). COX-2 plays an important role in causing inflammation throughout your body when it's activated by certain types of cells called mast cells--which are found throughout your skin surface area as well as other organs like joints where they release histamine when triggered by injury or other triggers like allergies or infections.

St. John's Wort

St. John's Wort, or Hypericum perforate, is a perennial herb with yellow flowers that grows in many parts of the world. The plant has been used for centuries to treat depression and anxiety. The name comes from the fact that it blooms around June 24th (St John's Day), which is when many other plants bloom as well--including Bugleweed (Ajuga reptant) and Woodruff (Asperula odorata).

St John's Wort has also been called Tipton's Weed, Klamath weed, and Goat weed because it was used by Native herbs who lived along rivers in Oregon; these people would collect leaves from these plants during springtime while they were still damp from rainstorms so they could make tea out of them later on when needed for medicinal purposes such as helping calm nerves or soothe sore throats.

Catnip

Catnip is a perennial herb that belongs to the mint family. It's native to Europe and Asia, but it grows well in North America as well.

Catnip has been used for centuries as a medicinal herb, as well as for its flavor and fragrance. It can be used in teas, tinctures, and tablets.

Fennel

Fennel is a great herb to use in cooking, as it adds an interesting flavor to dishes. It's also an excellent source of vitamin C, calcium, and iron- all three essential for good health. Fennel helps with digestion and bloating by promoting bile flow from the gallbladder; this helps break down fats and proteins so they can be absorbed into your body more easily.

Fennel seeds can also be chewed after a meal to help with heartburn or indigestion caused by overeating (or even eating too fast!).

Calendula

Calendula is a bright, cheerful herb that's great for skin and hair. It can also help with digestion and reduce inflammation. The flowers of calendula have been used to treat wounds, infections, eczema, and psoriasis for centuries--and modern science has confirmed that it does indeed have healing properties. Calendula floss (the Latin name for the flower) contains vitamins A and C, and powerful antioxidants called flavonoids that reduce free radical damage caused by pollution or sun exposure by scavenging them before they cause damage to your body tissues.

Comfrey

Comfrey is a perennial plant that grows in temperate climates. It has a long history of use in traditional medicine, and it's used to make infusions and ointments. Comfrey can be applied topically to treat wounds, burns, bruises, and sprains.

Yarrow

Yarrow is a hardy perennial that grows in sun or partial shade and thrives in dry soil. It's also known as milfoil, woundwort, and bloodwort--the latter because the leaves were used to staunch bleeding during battle. Yarrow has been used for centuries to treat infections and wounds; more recently, it's been used to treat fevers by Native herbs (who call it "bear medicine") as well as for digestive issues.

Nettle

Nettle is a common weed that grows in many places, and the leaves and stems can be used to make tea. The tea has diuretic and anti-inflammatory properties, which means it helps your body get rid of excess fluid (for example, if you have water retention). It's also used to treat urinary tract infections by increasing urine output.

Nettle leaf tea should not be taken by people with kidney disease or gout because it contains sodium that could worsen these conditions. If you've recently had surgery or have an enlarged prostate gland (prostate gland), talk with your doctor before drinking nettle leaf tea because it may cause irritation in these areas.

Flaxseed

Flaxseed is used for treating inflammation, arthritis, and gout. It can also be helpful in eczema, psoriasis, and scabies. Red clover has been shown to have an antibacterial effect on skin infections such as acne.

By now, you're probably ready to go out and try some of these herbs. But before you do, remember that it's important to talk with your doctor if you have any medical conditions or allergies. And remember: just because they're natural doesn't mean they're safe! Always use caution when using any herb or supplement--and never take more than what's recommended on the label without first consulting with someone who knows about its effects on the body.

Chapter 04 Benefits and Uses of Herbal Medicine

Herbal medicine is a form of alternative medicine that uses plants to help prevent and treat medical conditions. Humans have used many herbal remedies for thousands of years, but these days they aren't as popular as they once were. While some people still use herbal medicines today, they are not regulated by the Food and Drug Administration (FDA) like prescription or over-the-counter medications.

Humans have used medicinal plants for thousands of years.

Many of the medicines that we use today are derived from natural sources. For example, aspirin was first isolated from willow bark in 1838, and its active ingredient is silicon, which can be found in many other plants as well.

While there have been some advances in modern medicine, herbal remedies still play an important role in many cultures around the world today--and they may become even more important as we learn how to use them more effectively!

Herbs are not synthetic drugs.

Synthetic drugs are made in a laboratory and have no medicinal value, while herbs are naturally occurring plants or plant parts used for thousands of years by different cultures around the world as medicine.

Herbs may be used in combination with prescription medications.

This can help you get the best results from both therapies, and it's an option that many people prefer to avoid taking synthetic drugs.

Herbal medicine is not a substitute for conventional medical treatment but can be used as an adjunct to complement your doctor's recommendations.

Herbs may interact with prescription medications or other supplements you are taking.

Before using herbs, tell your doctor if you are taking any prescription drugs, including blood thinners such as warfarin (Coumadin); drugs for high blood pressure; drugs for diabetes; steroids; heart medicines such as digoxin (Lanoxin); seizure medications such as phenytoin (Dilantin) and carbamazepine (Tegretol); anti-inflammatory drugs such as aspirin and ibuprofen (Advil); birth control pills; antibiotics such as amoxicillin or tetracycline; antifungal medication such as ketoconazole cream; cancer chemotherapy drugs like cyclophosphamide and cisplatin.

Herbal medicine offers many benefits and uses.

The following are some of the most common:

- It's a safe, natural alternative to conventional medicine. Herbals can be used as an adjunct to conventional medical treatment or as a standalone treatment option, depending on your circumstances and preferences.
- They're inexpensive compared to prescription drugs or over-the-counter medications (though they may not be covered by insurance). Some herbs also grow wild in your backyard or can be harvested from your garden!

Herbal medicine can help with minor health issues such as headaches, colds, and digestive problems.

Most herbal medicines work in three ways: stimulating the immune system, killing or preventing the growth of bacteria or viruses (antibiotics), or soothing inflammation (anti-inflammatory).

Herbal medicine can help with chronic health issues and may even be used as a replacement for prescribed medication.

- Hereunto: This supplement is made up of herbs that the Chinese have used for thousands of years to treat digestive issues such as bloating, constipation, and diarrhea. It also helps to improve liver function by supporting healthy bile production, which helps you digest fats more efficiently and absorb nutrients from your food better.
- Resourceful Medicine: This product contains 14 different herbs that work together to support healthy blood pressure levels while lowering cholesterol levels. It's good for people with high blood pressure- it can also lower your risk of developing hypertension later in life!

However, herbal medicine is not recommended for people who have serious medical conditions or are taking prescription medications. Herbs can interact with other drugs and cause dangerous effects. Talk to your doctor first if you're concerned about how your herbal product might interact with other medicines

.

Suppose you have a severe illness or take prescription drugs on a regular basis. In that case, it's best to avoid using herbal remedies altogether until you've spoken with a qualified healthcare provider about your situation and decided whether they are right for you.

Herbal medicine is a form of alternative medicine that uses plants to help prevent and treat medical conditions. Herbal medicines have been used since ancient times, with evidence of their use in China dating back 5,000 years.

Herbs are often sold as dietary supplements at health food stores and online, but trained practitioners can also prepare them as teas, tinctures, and salves (a thick lotion).

Many herbal medicines are derived from plants- some medicinal or poisonous. Although most people think of herbs as the leaves and flowers of plants, they actually include any parts of a plant that can be used to heal disease or treat symptoms.

Drinks made from herbs were popular remedies in America during the colonial era.

People believed that certain herbal teas had healing powers and drank them to help with various health problems. Some of these drinks are still used today as natural medicines.

The popularity of herbal medicine grew during the 19th century, and many people used it without consulting doctors or other medical professionals. This can be seen in Samuel Thomson's work, which published his book

The New Guide to Health in 1822. The book was widely read by farmers and homemakers who wanted to learn how to treat themselves using herbs and other ingredients that were readily available on their property.

In the early 20th century, with the rise of pharmaceutical drugs and their promise of quick fixes, people often stopped using herbal remedies. However, this is not to say that they have completely gone away. There are still many places around the world where herbal medicine remains a viable option for treating illnesses and injuries. Some modern medical practitioners use herbs alongside their pharmaceuticals to treat patients' ailments integratively (that is, combining both types of treatment).

Today, interest in herbal medicine is growing again thanks to its purported benefits.

Herbalists claim that herbs are effective at treating a wide variety of ailments and can also be used as preventatives for certain conditions.

Herbs have been used throughout history as part of traditional medicine.

Herbal Medications can be helpful but should be used with caution

Herbs have been used for thousands of years to treat various health conditions. While herbal medicines can be helpful, they should be used with caution. The following are some reasons why:

- Herbs are not regulated by the Food and Drug Administration (FDA).
- The potency and purity of herbs can vary greatly from one brand to another.
- Herbs interact with other medications you may be taking, so it's important to talk with your doctor before starting an herbal supplement program.

Herbal medicine is the use of herbs for health.

Herbalists use a variety of plants and plant extracts in their practice, including flowers, leaves, seeds, roots, or berries. "Herb" refers to plants with little or no secondary growth (woody stems). They are also known as "soft plants."

Herbs have been used for thousands of years by humans across many cultures around the world; some examples include Ayurveda in India; Traditional Chinese Medicine (TCM) in China; Unani Tibbs System in Pakistan; Siddha Medicine System in South India; Jamu Traditional Medicine System - Indonesia.

Herbalists make natural remedies using different techniques, such as drying out plant parts and using them later or extracting certain compounds from plants to create medicinal products.

Herbal medicine can be used alone or with other treatments like traditional Chinese medicine (TCM), homeopathy, or Ayurveda.

Some herbal medicines work better when combined with other foods or herbs.

Herbs can be used alone or combined with other foods. Herbs are sometimes used in combination with other herbs to treat specific conditions, such as the following:

- Garlic and ginger have been shown to reduce blood pressure when taken together.
- If you have high blood pressure or diabetes, try taking garlic with rosemary and oregano (two herbs known for their ability to lower blood sugar).

Herbal medicine can be used alone (for simple conditions) or in combination with prescription drugs (in the case of serious conditions). For example, your doctor may prescribe antibiotics if you have an infection. However, herbal remedies like turmeric or ginger can also help fight off infections and reduce inflammation in your body.

Herbs are often used as part of a holistic approach to health care that focuses on treating the whole person rather than just symptoms. This means that when choosing an herbal supplement for yourself or loved ones--even children!--it's important to consider what ailment needs healing and whether any underlying causes of illness might benefit from additional treatment such as lifestyle changes or dietary changes.

Herbal supplements are not regulated by the Food and Drug Administration (FDA), although they are considered foods rather than drugs or medications. The FDA does not review herbal supplements before being sold to consumers; manufacturers must ensure that their products are safe before putting them on store shelves.

Herbal medicine is a form of alternative medicine that uses plants, herbs, and other natural sources to treat medical conditions. Herbalism has been practiced for thousands of years around the world, with evidence dating back to ancient Egypt and China.

It's important to note that the Food & Drug Administration (FDA) does not regulate herbal medicines. You can't always trust what you read on an herbal product label because this agency sets no standards.

Herbal medicine has been used for thousands of years, from treating chronic conditions to minor ailments.

You might have heard about the ancient practice of using plants and herbs to treat various illnesses, but what exactly is herbal medicine?

Herbs are often used in combination with other types of treatments. For example, herbal medicine may be used to treat symptoms of depression and anxiety, but you'll likely also need to go to therapy or take medication if your condition is severe.

Herbal medicine is safe and natural.

The herbs used in herbal medicine have been used for thousands of years, and they're grown organically with no pesticides or other harmful chemicals. Herbalists believe that the body's energy systems can be strengthened through herbs, which help to balance your emotions and mind so you feel better overall.

Herbal remedies are made from plants that grow naturally in different parts of the world. These herbs have always been used by people who live close to nature--they know what works best!

Herbalism is a cost-effective alternative to conventional medicine, using herbs as its main ingredients. The cost of herbal remedies varies depending on the type and brand you buy, but it's generally much lower than conventional drugs that contain chemicals or synthetic substances.

There may be some interactions with other medications.

Because herbal medicines are plant-based, some interactions with other medications may occur. For example, if you are taking blood pressure medication and also want to take an herbal remedy for your high blood pressure (hypertension), it's important that you talk to your doctor first.

If you have any questions or concerns about using herbal remedies alongside other health products or treatments, always speak with a qualified healthcare professional.

Some herbs are harmful and can even be deadly when taken on their own.

Some herbs can be harmful if taken on their own. For example, skullcap and lobelia are two herbs that can cause seizures when taken in large doses. Pine bark extract is another example of an herb that can be dangerous if you don't know what you're doing; it's been linked to liver damage when taken without proper supervision. If you're going to use herbal medicine as part of your treatment plan, consult with a professional beforehand so they can guide you through any potential risks or side effects before starting any kind of treatment plan based on these natural remedies.

Herbal medicine is useful and safe, but knowing what you're getting into is important before you try it.

Herbs or parts of plants have been used in traditional medicine for centuries. They can be eaten, brewed into tea, or used topically (on the skin). Herbs have many uses: they may help digestion, relieve pain and reduce inflammation. Some are also used as natural alternatives to prescription drugs because they act like chemicals found in these drugs but without side effects or risk of addiction.

The use of herbs has been around since ancient times.

The first recorded use of herbs was in China over 5000 years ago. The ancient Greeks used them as well, and they have continued to be used throughout history by many cultures around the world.

Herbs are used to treat a variety of different ailments and conditions.

The use of herbs dates back to ancient times and was used by many civilizations for various ailments and conditions. Herbs were not just limited to humans; they were also used on animals like horses or livestock.

Herbal medicine has been a part of our history for thousands of years, but recently its popularity has been resurgent because of scientific studies confirming its effectiveness.

Doctors often prescribe medications that contain synthetic chemicals instead of using herbs because they believe those medications are safer than natural ones, like those found in herbal products made from plants or trees. However, these synthetic drugs have side effects that may be worse than taking nothing at all!

Natural remedies can be made at home.

This is a great way to save money and ensure you get a natural product. Here are some of the most common ingredients used in herbal remedies:

- Comfrey leaves - for bruises, sprains, and swelling
- Chamomile flowers - for digestive problems such as bloating or indigestion

Some common herbs include chamomile, peppermint, echinacea, and ginger root.

These can be used to help with things like diarrhea or stomach pain and to treat colds.

Herbs are also good for making your own beauty products, such as face masks or lotions that you can use on your skin. They have natural ingredients that will make your skin look healthy and soft!

Herbal medicine has a long history and many uses.

Herbalism is the use of plants, their extracts, and other natural products (such as bee pollen) to prevent or treat disease. The word herbal comes from the Latin herbal, meaning "plant." Herbs have been used for thousands of years by ancient cultures around the world for their medicinal properties.

Medicinal plants have been used for thousands of years.

Many herbal remedies are still used today, although they may be less well-known than conventional drugs. Herbal medicine can be safe and effective if you use it correctly.

- It can also be used as a preventative measure against illness by boosting the immune system.
- Herbal medicines may be taken in tablet form or as infusions (teas) made from dried herbs that have been crushed into small pieces or powdered into a powder form.

Herbal remedies often use plant extracts that contain natural chemicals that help fight disease.

These chemicals are called phytochemicals and can be found in many plants, including:

- Turmeric (Curcuma longa)
- Cinnamon (Cinnamomum verum)
- Black pepper (Piper nigrum)

These herbs have been used for centuries to treat diseases, including cancer, diabetes, and heart disease.

Some herbs may work better when combined with other vitamins or minerals.

Herbs can be used on their own or in combination with other herbs, vitamins, and minerals. When you're trying to get better from an illness or disease, your doctor needs to know about everything you take.

When using herbal medicine, it's important to consult a doctor before taking any supplement because of possible interactions with other medications.

Some herbs can be taken safely on their own and others should only be used under the supervision of an expert.

Using natural remedies is a great way to treat some common illnesses without spending a lot of money on medications.

Natural remedies are also safer than conventional drugs since they don't have side effects and can be used by people with sensitive bodies or allergies.

Herbal medicine is an alternative medicine that uses plants and plant extracts.

It's been used for thousands of years to treat many health conditions, including pain, stress, and digestive problems. Herbal products are available in many forms, including teas, tablets, or capsules that you can buy online or at health food stores. They may also be sold as creams or oils applied directly to the skin.

Herbal medicine is used to treat everything from headaches to heart disease.

The ancient art of herbalism can be traced back more than 5,000 years and has been practiced in many parts of the world, including China and India. Today, herbal medicine is gaining popularity as an alternative treatment for many health conditions because it's natural and doesn't have side effects like prescription drugs. Herbs or parts of plants have been used for medicinal purposes since ancient times. They contain chemical compounds that may help prevent or treat certain health problems when taken internally (eaten), applied topically (applied onto the skin), or inhaled as steam vapors through teas or poultices.

Herbal medicine can be an effective way to treat certain medical conditions.

The use of herbs for medicinal purposes dates back thousands of years, and many cultures have used them to treat various ailments. Today, herbalism is a popular alternative health practice that focuses on the use of plants and their extracts as remedies for both physical and emotional disorders.

Herbs have been used throughout history to treat both acute and chronic conditions such as heart disease, depression, and anxiety disorders (1). They've also been shown to help with pain management (2). Herbalists may use a variety of herbs for different reasons: some act as stimulants while others are sedatives; some promote relaxation while others calm an overactive mind; some reduce inflammation while others reduce pain in muscles or joints through anti-inflammatory properties

Many possible side effects are associated with herbal medicines, including severe allergic reactions.

One of the most important things to remember when using herbal medicine is that there are many possible side effects, including severe allergic reactions. If you're taking any kind of medication or supplement and have a reaction to it, stop using it immediately and contact your doctor or medical professional.

If you experience any unusual symptoms after using herbal medicines, or if your condition worsens, contact your doctor.

Herbal medicine can be an alternative to conventional medicine, and it's important to understand how they both work. Herbs have been used for thousands of years as part of traditional medicine systems around the world. Many of these herbs are still used today as part of modern medicine, even if we don't always realize it!

Herbs can be used in many ways: some are taken orally (eaten), and others are applied topically (on your skin). Some herbs are used internally, while others are used externally. The most common way to use herbs is through tea--you may have heard about chamomile or ginger tea before!

PART 02

Chapter 05 Natural Herbal Remedies

If you're looking for natural herbal remedies, herbalists have been using them for centuries. Herbal remedies can be used to treat a wide range of health issues, including colds and flu, heartburn and digestive problems, muscle pain, and insomnia. Some herbal remedies are even known to help fight cancer or prevent diabetes.

Herbal medicine is a branch of traditional medicine that uses plant extracts as primary therapy. Herbs have been used for thousands of years and are still used today. There are many different types of herbal medicine, and the active ingredients in herbal medicine are called phytochemicals. Herbal medicines can be used to treat or prevent disease or taken to improve general health. This chapter will examine how herbal medicine works and some clinical studies showing its effectiveness as an anti-inflammatory agent.

- Turmeric is a powerful anti-inflammatory agent that's been used in Eastern medicine for centuries. It contains curcumin, which has been shown to help relieve joint pain and reduce swelling.

- Turmeric may be one of the most potent anti-inflammatory herbs out there!

- Turmeric, a spice used in Indian cuisine, contains curcumin. Curcumin is the most common active ingredient in turmeric, and research suggests it can help reduce joint pain related to osteoarthritis.

- Curcumin is so effective at easing joint inflammation that it outperforms common drugs like ibuprofen and aspirin in clinical trials.

- A study published in the Journal of Alternative Complementary Medicine found that curcumin could reduce pain by 32% within two hours of consumption--and this wasn't just a short-term reduction; participants reported continued relief for up to 24 hours after taking the supplement.

- Curcumin's anti-inflammatory properties also make it a promising treatment for rheumatoid arthritis, Crohn's disease, and other inflammatory disorders.

- In one study published in Arthritis Research & Therapy, researchers gave curcumin to patients with rheumatoid arthritis. They found it reduced joint pain and stiffness after three months of treatment.

Turmeric is one of the most well-known herbs in the world. It's been used for thousands of years in Ayurvedic medicine and as a spice in cooking. Turmeric has also been shown to have anti-inflammatory properties that may help reduce symptoms of several inflammatory conditions, including:

- Arthritis (rheumatoid)
- Asthma
- Crohn's disease

Turmeric is thought to work by inhibiting COX enzymes--the same ones targeted by nonsteroidal anti-inflammatory drugs (NSAIDs).

Herbal medicine is a branch of traditional medicine that uses plant extracts as primary therapy. It has been practiced for thousands of years and relies on the use of plants with medicinal properties to treat disease.

The goal of herbal medicine is to cure diseases without side effects.

You may be wondering why there are so many herbal medicines. The reason is that herbal medicine can cure diseases without side effects, which is what we all want when we're sick. It's also important to note that these herbs are natural and don't contain any chemicals or preservatives.

Herbal medicine has been used for thousands of years and is still used today.

Herbal medicine is a type of alternative medicine that uses plant-based chemicals as the main treatment. Herbs can be taken as food or drink or applied directly to the skin in ointments or oils (called tinctures).

There are many studies on herbal medicine, but there are still many questions about them.

Herbal medicine is the use of plant-derived materials, such as leaves and roots. They can be used internally (eaten) or externally (topically).

One study showed that ginkgo biloba had an anti-inflammatory effect.

In this study, researchers compared the effects of ginkgo biloba (GB) with those of celecoxib, a prescription medication used to treat inflammation and pain associated with arthritis. The results revealed that GB was just as effective as celecoxib in reducing symptoms such as swelling and tenderness; however, it did not cause any side effects such as nausea or diarrhea--two common side effects associated with celecoxib use.

The use of herbal medicine dates back to prehistoric times.

Herbal medicine has been used for thousands of years. The first recorded use of herbs dates back to prehistoric times, when the human race began to develop agriculture and use plants for food and medicine. In ancient Greece, Hippocrates (460-370 BC) wrote about the healing properties of various plants; in China, Shen Nong (2600 BC) developed an extensive system of herbal medicine that was later codified by Li Shenzhen (1518-1593).

More recently, herbal remedies were popularized by Europeans who traveled around the world collecting "exotic" herbs and spices from faraway lands. These were often used as ingredients in cooking or as medicines at home but did not gain widespread acceptance until they were standardized into pills or powders that could be easily administered without much preparation required on behalf of patients.

There are many different types of herbal medicine.

The most common are:

- Herbal teas can be made from leaves, flowers, and other parts of plants. They're often used to make infusions or decoctions (a strong-tasting drink).
- Tinctures (also called extracts) are made by soaking herbs in alcohol for several weeks before straining out the liquid. Tinctures have been used as medicine since ancient times because they're easy to carry around and take with you when you travel or go on long journeys away from home.
- The active ingredients in herbal medicine are called phytochemicals.
- These plant-based chemicals have antioxidant and anti-inflammatory properties, which make them good for your health.

Herbal medicine is less expensive than conventional drugs.

Herbal medicines are manufactured from plants, which are grown all over the world and have been used for thousands of years by people in different cultures. They don't require expensive laboratory testing or large-scale manufacturing processes, so they tend to be much cheaper than prescription medications and over-the-counter drugs.

Herbal medicines can be used to treat or prevent disease or taken to improve general health. Herbal medicines may have some side effects and interactions with other medications. Some herbal products are not regulated by the U.S. Food and Drug Administration (FDA).

Many traditional healers use herbal medicine as a way to improve overall well-being.

This type of treatment is often used to address the root cause of a problem rather than just treating the symptoms. For example, suppose you have an infection in your throat caused by bacteria. In that case, a doctor may prescribe antibiotics to kill off those bacteria so they no longer cause problems. However, suppose you are suffering from an underlying condition that causes inflammation (such as Crohn's disease). In that case, antibiotics will not help because they do not address the underlying cause. Herbal remedies can be used instead because they have anti-inflammatory properties, which reduce swelling and pain caused by inflammation within cells or tissues throughout our bodies.

Traditional medicine has long been used in both Western and Eastern cultures.

This can be traced back to the ancient Greeks, who were among the first to recognize the importance of plant-based remedies. As time went on and technology advanced, these practices were replaced by modern medicine-- but now there's a growing interest in traditional healing methods again.

Traditional herbal remedies are still widely used today because they're considered safe and effective for treating many conditions without side effects. They're also often less expensive than prescription drugs or other treatments that may require frequent visits to your doctor or hospital!

Aromatherapy is a form of alternative medicine that uses the aromatic compounds of plants to improve health, including stress reduction and the treatment of various physical conditions. It's based on the idea that smells influence our moods and emotions.

Aromatherapy was developed in France during World War I as an aid for soldiers suffering from shell shock, but it wasn't until after World War II that it gained popularity among civilians. Today, aromatherapists use essential oils extracted from flowers or leaves; these can be applied directly to the skin (such as with massage), inhaled through steam baths or diffusers, or added to other products such as soap or lotion.

Ayurvedic medicine is an ancient Indian natural medicine system developed over thousands of years. It focuses on healing the whole person and not just the symptoms of a disease.

Ayurvedic doctors believe that health depends on a balance between body, mind, and spirit. They treat each patient individually to restore this balance through diet changes or herbal remedies depending on their constitution (Prakriti).

Homeopathy is a medical philosophy that all conditions are treatable with small, highly diluted amounts of natural substances that cause similar symptoms in healthy people. The practice was developed by German physician Samuel Hahnemann in 1796 and has since been used to treat a wide variety of ailments.

Hahnemann believed water could retain the memory of substances it had once contained, even after being boiled or filtered, so he began diluting his medications until none remained--a process known as potentization or succussion (Suk-sash-shun). In this way, homeopathic remedies are not made from plants or minerals but instead consist solely of their energetic imprints on water molecules found at their original concentrations within nature's matrixes.

Herbal treatments can be used to treat many common ailments.

Herbs are plants that grow naturally and have been used for centuries as medicine by many cultures. Herbs have been found to be effective in treating a variety of illnesses, including arthritis and high blood pressure.

One way to use herbs is by making them into a tea or tincture.

Throw the herbs in boiling water for 10 minutes to make an herbal tea. Strain out the herbs and drink it hot or cold. You can also add honey if you like it sweeter!

For making tinctures (alcohol extracts), put 1 cup of dried herb material into a mason jar with 1 cup of vodka or brandy for every ounce of herb material used (for example, if you're using two tablespoons of dried stinging nettle leaves, then use 16 ounces) and seal tightly with cheesecloth over the top so no bugs get in there while they sit on your shelf for at least 4 weeks before straining out all plant matter using cheesecloth again (or muslin cloth).

Herbs can help reduce inflammation and pain by acting on different targets in the body to reduce inflammation. Some herbs have anti-inflammatory properties that work by inhibiting COX-1 and COX-2 enzymes. These two enzymes are responsible for producing prostaglandins, which play a role in causing inflammation and pain.

Herbal medicine is a traditional medicine used for thousands of years. It is still widely practiced today, and many different types of herbal medicine exist. Herbs can treat or prevent disease and improve general health by reducing inflammation and pain.

Tribulus

Tribulus is a plant that has been used for centuries in traditional medicine. It's been used to treat sexual problems, infertility, and symptoms of menopause and PMS.

Tribulus can help with weight loss by increasing metabolism, improving energy levels, and reducing cravings for high-fat foods.

Skullcap

Skullcap, a perennial herb with a bitter taste and a slight peppermint scent, is used as a sedative and anti-inflammatory. It's also used for insomnia, anxiety, and muscle spasms.

Rho Diola

Rho Diola is a perennial herb that grows in cold, arctic climates and is native to Europe, Asia, and North America. It's been used for centuries in Eastern Europe and Scandinavia as a tonic herb. The plant's root has been shown to help alleviate depression by increasing serotonin levels in the brain.

Rho Diola also has antioxidant properties that may protect against free radicals (cells that damage other cells). This can help prevent cell damage from radiation therapy or chemotherapy treatments for cancer patients who want to reduce their risk of complications from these therapies.

Maca

Maca root has a long history of use as a medicinal herb. It's been used for thousands of years in the Andes Mountains of Peru, Chile, and Bolivia to treat various health issues and boost energy levels.

Maca is an adaptogen that can help your body adapt to stress by balancing hormones (like cortisol), improving cognitive function and mood, boosting libido, increasing fertility rates in women, reducing cholesterol levels in menopausal women who are at risk for heart disease--and that's just scratching the surface!

Evening Primrose

Evening primrose is a common plant that grows throughout the world. It has been used for centuries to treat various conditions, including depression and anxiety. The leaves of evening primrose contain an essential oil that helps regulate hormone levels in your body and reduce inflammation.

It's best to take evening primrose oil orally as opposed to applying it directly on skin or wounds because its effects are more potent when absorbed into the bloodstream through digestion rather than applied topically (through your mouth).

Kava

Kava is a natural herbal remedy that can help you relax and sleep better. It's not recommended for pregnant women, people with liver problems, or people taking certain medications.

Kava has been a traditional medicine in the Pacific Islands for centuries. Some studies have shown that kava may be helpful in treating anxiety disorders such as generalized anxiety disorder (GAD), social phobia, panic attacks, and post-traumatic stress disorder (PTSD).

Black Cohosh

Black cohosh is an estrogenic herb that can help balance female hormones. It's used to treat menopause symptoms like hot flashes and night sweats. Black cohosh has also been shown to be effective for osteoarthritis and rheumatoid arthritis--it may help relieve joint pain, stiffness, or swelling.

Black cohosh should not be used during pregnancy because it could cause premature birth, miscarriage, or even death of the fetus if taken in large doses (more than two cups per day).

Holy Basil

This herb is a great stress reliever, and it can help with insomnia, anxiety, depression and headaches. It's also been used to treat indigestion and colds/flu (when combined with other herbs).

Turmeric Extracts and Powders

Turmeric, or curcumin, is a good anti-inflammatory and antioxidant. It can be used for arthritis, joint pain, and other inflammatory conditions. Turmeric has been shown to reduce symptoms of osteoarthritis by as much as 50 percent in just 3 months!

Turmeric can be taken in capsule form or as a powder mixed with water (1 tablespoon of turmeric powder per cup of water).

These herbs can help you prevent illness, manage pain and boost your immune system.

Many herbs have been used for centuries to treat a variety of ailments and medical conditions. Herbs can help you prevent illness, manage pain and boost your immune system.

Some common herbs include:

- Chamomile - Chamomile tea is known for its calming effects on the body. It can be used as a sleep aid or herbal tea to relax after a long day at work or school. You can also use it as an herbal bath to soothe sore muscles after working out at the gym!
- Echinacea - This herb has been shown in studies to boost the immune system when taken regularly over time (about two weeks). It's great if you're going through cold/flu season because it will help keep those germs away from you!

Aloe Vera Gel

Aloe vera gel is a natural remedy that can be used to treat many ailments. It's best known for its ability to relieve burns, cuts, and sunburns, but it also has other uses.

Aloe vera gel can be applied directly to the skin as an acne treatment; it's also effective at helping psoriasis sufferers keep their condition under control by reducing inflammation and redness caused by their condition. The plant's juice has been found to be effective in treating dandruff when applied externally or consumed internally (in the form of aloe vera juice).

Cinnamon

Cinnamon is a traditional remedy for colds and flu. It can help boost your immune system, making it a smart choice when feeling under the weather. Cinnamon can be consumed in food and drink or taken as a supplement, but it also works topically on skin infections like acne and athlete's foot.

Chamomile Tea

Chamomile tea is an herbal remedy that's been used for centuries to treat a variety of health conditions. It can be prepared from the dried flowers of chamomile plants, which are often blended with other ingredients such as mint or ginger. Drinking this tea includes relieving stress and anxiety, improving sleep quality, and reducing inflammation and pain symptoms associated with arthritis (1).

To make chamomile tea at home:

- Boil water in a kettle or saucepan until it reaches boiling point (212 degrees F). Pour 3 cups into a teapot or heat-proof pitcher and add 1 tablespoon of dried chamomile flowers per cupful of water. Steep for 10 minutes before straining out any loose-leaf matter using a fine mesh strainer lined with cheesecloth if desired.

Cat's Claw

Cat's claw is a vine that grows in the Amazon rainforest. The plant has been used to treat gastrointestinal and respiratory problems and inflammation. Cat's claw contains active compounds that have anti-inflammatory properties, which make it an effective treatment for joint pain, arthritis, and other inflammatory diseases.

Cat's claw has been used by the people of the Amazon for centuries to treat various ailments, including acute diarrhea (especially when caused by parasites), intestinal worm infections, and arthritis pain.

Apple cider vinegar

Apple cider vinegar is a natural remedy for fighting colds and the flu. It can be used in salad dressings, marinades, and sauces. You can also use it as a hair rinse, skin toner, or to help treat acne.

Apple cider vinegar has been around for hundreds of years and has many uses besides being an ingredient in your favorite salad dressing!

Castor oil

Castor oil is a popular remedy for constipation. It can be taken orally or used topically on the skin to treat acne and psoriasis. Castor oil also has laxative properties, so it can be taken in small amounts to relieve constipation.

Epsom salt baths

Epsom salt baths are a great way to relax and relieve stress. To get the most out of your Epsom salt bath, you'll want to use about a cup of Epsom salt in lukewarm water. The best time for an Epsom salt bath is when you're feeling tired or stressed after work or school.

Make sure that the water is not too hot for your skin--you should be able to comfortably hold your hand under it without burning yourself (but don't try this at home!). Pour some Epsom salts into your tub and any other essential oils or fragrances you'd like added to the mix. You can also add bath bombs if they're available at your local store; these will help soften up any rough patches on your skin while making sure that everything smells nice!

When finished soaking, make sure not only not to towel off immediately but also to pat dry instead--this will help lock in moisture which leads us directly to our next tip:

Essential oils

Essential oils are made from the aromatic parts of plants and contain their natural healing properties. They can be used for aromatherapy, massage, and other applications. Essential oils can also be used for a variety of ailments, including headaches and stress relief.

Essential oils should never be taken internally without guidance from a qualified professional because they may cause harm if not used properly or in the right amount.

Garlic

Garlic is a natural antibiotic and immune booster. It's also been shown to have anti-inflammatory properties, as well as being able to reduce pain and swelling in the body.

The active ingredient in garlic that makes it so effective is allicin, which has been shown to destroy harmful bacteria like E. coli and staph infections. Garlic also contains selenium, which helps boost the immune system by increasing white blood cell count (a type of infection-fighting cell).

Honey

Honey is a natural sweetener that can be used to treat coughs and sore throats. It also has anti-inflammatory properties, which can help heal wounds, burns, and other skin issues like acne.

Lemon juice

Lemon juice is one of the most effective natural skin lighteners. It can be used to remove dark spots and prevent stretch marks, pimples, and scars.

73

Lemon juice has anti-aging properties that help reduce wrinkles and fine lines on your face. It also helps fight acne by killing bacteria, drying out excess oil in your pores, exfoliating dead skin cells, and reducing inflammation caused by blemishes.

Natural remedies are both affordable and healthy.

Natural remedies are often cheaper than medications. While they may not be as effective at treating medical conditions, they can be used as an alternative or supplement to pharmaceuticals.

Natural remedies are also healthier than medications because they do not have the same side effects that drugs have, such as nausea and dizziness.

In addition to being safe and effective, natural remedies can help you save money on your healthcare expenses by reducing how often you need to see a doctor for treatment of minor illnesses such as colds and flu.

Chamomile tea

Chamomile tea is a calming and relaxing drink that can help you sleep, relieve menstrual cramps, and even aid digestion. It's also been known to ease skin irritation, allergies, and colds and coughs.

Lavender oil

Lavender oil is a popular essential oil that can be used for many different ailments. It has been used for centuries as a natural remedy for a wide range of illnesses, including:

- Insomnia and anxiety
- Acne and eczema
- Headaches and migraines

Peppermint essential oil

Peppermint essential oil is a natural antispasmodic, which means it helps to relax tense muscles and relieve stress and anxiety. It can also be used to improve digestion, reduce nausea, or reduce inflammation.

Yarrow

Yarrow is an herb that has been used for centuries to treat wounds and infections. It contains a chemical compound called "achilleate," which has been shown to help fight bacteria, fungi, and viruses.

Achillean is present in the leaves of yarrow but not the flowers or stems. If you're using fresh herbs (not dried), make sure to harvest those parts separately so that you don't include any other parts of the plant in your remedy!

Yarrow can be applied directly to cuts or scrapes as a poultice - just crush up some leaves with water until they form a paste and apply this directly onto your wound/scratch area for 10 minutes at a time until it heals completely (about 24 hours). You can also drink 1-2 cups every day as well if desired--this will strengthen your immune system so that any colds/flu viruses try attacking them first before getting anywhere near our bodies' vital organs!

Slippery Elm

Slippery Elm is an herb that is used to treat inflammation and diarrhea. It is also used to treat sore throats and chest congestion caused by colds and flu. Slippery Elm can be used for digestive problems like heartburn, indigestion, or ulcers.

Ginger root

Ginger root is a powerful anti-inflammatory and natural pain reliever. It can be used to treat arthritis, muscle pain, and sore throats. Ginger is also an excellent natural remedy for nausea (including morning sickness), motion sickness, and headaches.

Ginger has long been used in Ayurvedic medicine as well as Chinese traditional medicine (TCM). In TCM, it's believed that ginger helps reduce heat or fire energy in the body, which may cause symptoms such as fever or hot flashes during menopause.

Saw Palmetto

Saw palmetto is a natural herbal remedy that can help with prostate enlargement, urinary tract infections, and other conditions. It is available in capsule form and can be used to treat urinary tract infections. Saw palmetto is also used to treat prostate enlargement.

Apple cider vinegar

Apple cider vinegar is a natural detoxifier that can help you lose weight and lower cholesterol. It's also a remedy for heartburn, high blood pressure, diabetes and allergies.

Apple cider vinegar is made from apple juice (usually unpasteurized). The fermentation process produces acetic acid, which gives vinegar its sour taste. Most of the time, you'll find it in liquid form, but there are also capsules available if you prefer to take them instead of drinking them!

Honey

Honey is a natural moisturizer that can be used to treat acne. It's antibacterial and antifungal, making it great for the treatment of acne-prone skin. In addition to its anti-inflammatory properties, honey is also a humectant--it attracts moisture to your skin! This makes it an especially effective treatment for dehydrated skin types.

Honey has been shown to have antioxidant properties as well, which means it helps protect against free radical damage caused by UV exposure (which leads to wrinkles).

Red Clover

Red clover is a flowering plant native to Europe, Asia, and North America. It's also used to make medicine. Red clover has been used for thousands of years to treat stomach problems such as ulcers and irritable bowel syndrome (IBS). Today it's sometimes used as an alternative treatment for cancer by people who don't want to take radiation or chemotherapy drugs because they can have serious side effects like hair loss or nausea.

Red clover contains chemicals called phytoestrogens that may help block the effects of estrogen in your body--which could be helpful if you're having trouble getting pregnant because you have low levels of estrogen during menopause (the stage when women stop having periods). However, there isn't enough research yet about how effective red clover is at treating infertility caused by low estrogen levels.

Cilantro, parsley, and oregano (for cooking)

Cilantro, parsley, and oregano are great natural herbs to have in your kitchen. They can help fight illnesses by boosting your immune system and keeping you healthy.

- Cilantro: Cilantro is rich in antioxidants that help fight inflammation, making it a good choice for people with arthritis or other joint problems. It's also a natural diuretic that can reduce bloating associated with water retention.
- Parsley: This herb is loaded with vitamins A and C as well as iron, potassium, and calcium--all nutrients that contribute to better overall health! Parsley helps to boost metabolism while also fighting free radicals (those nasty little guys who damage our cells) by neutralizing them before they do any damage!

These are some natural herbal remedies that have been used for centuries.

- Chamomile is an herb used for thousands of years as a sedative, anti-inflammatory and antispasmodic agent. It can be taken internally to treat insomnia, anxiety, and irritable bowel syndrome (IBS) or externally as a compress on bruises or sprains.
- Marshmallow root has been used since ancient times to treat upset stomachs, ulcers, and other gastrointestinal problems such as colitis and Crohn's disease by soothing inflamed tissue in the digestive tract while easing irritability or spasms caused by IBS symptoms like diarrhea or constipation.
- You should not use marshmallows if you have an allergy to ragweed pollen because it may cause an allergic reaction similar to hay fever symptoms such as sneezing or runny nose.

Eucalyptus oil

Eucalyptus oil is a great disinfectant that can treat respiratory problems such as coughs, colds, and flu. The oil also helps to clear blocked sinuses.

It can be used in the bath or as a massage oil if you have sore muscles, aches, and pains.

Tea tree oil

Tea tree oil is a natural antiseptic that can be used to treat acne and dandruff. Tea tree oil has anti-inflammatory properties, and it helps to reduce redness and swelling in the skin.

If you want to try tea tree oil for yourself, mix 1/2 teaspoon of lavender oil with 2 tablespoons of water until the mixture is completely dissolved. Then add 10 drops of tea tree oil (or more if necessary). Apply this mixture on your scalp every night before going to bed or after showering in the morning, massaging gently into dry hair until all parts are covered with liquid from head to toe, if possible!

Nettle Leaf

Nettle leaf is a natural remedy that has been used for centuries to treat a variety of ailments. It's an extract from the common stinging nettle plant and can be used to treat arthritis, eczema, psoriasis, and other skin conditions.

It also has anti-inflammatory properties, which can help reduce swelling in joints or muscles.

Lemon juice

Lemon juice is a great way to add flavor and nutrients to your food. You can:

- Add lemon juice to your water or other beverages.
- Use it as salad dressing, for example, with olive oil and salt.
- Marinate fish or chicken in it before cooking (the acid helps tenderize).
- Mix with rice or potatoes when baking them (great for flavor!).

And if you're not much of a cook, try adding some lemon juice into pasta sauces--it adds zing without changing the taste too much!

Marshmallow Root

Marshmallow root is a soothing herb that can be used to treat digestive issues and sore throats. It also has anti-inflammatory properties, which makes it beneficial for people who have been exposed to radiation.

This flowering plant contains compounds called saponins that make up about 10% of the root's weight. These compounds have several health benefits, including:

- Soothing effects on the digestive tract (it's often used as an herbal remedy for colitis)
- Anti-inflammatory properties (the saponins in marshmallow root help reduce swelling by preventing white blood cells from attaching themselves to tissues)

Licorice Root

Licorice root is an anti-inflammatory herb that can be used to treat acne and other skin problems. It's been used for centuries as a natural remedy and can also treat heartburn, stomach ulcers, and even cancer.

Licorice root extract contains chemicals called glycyrrhizin that have been shown in studies to reduce symptoms of psoriasis by reducing inflammation of the skin. In fact, one study found that licorice root helped people with moderate-to-severe plaque psoriasis improve their symptoms after only two weeks.

Licorice root may also help protect against sun damage on your face or body by helping block ultraviolet radiation from reaching deeper layers of your skin (3). This can reduce signs of premature aging, such as wrinkles around the eyes due to exposure from being outside for too long without sunscreen!

Ginseng

Ginseng is a plant that has been used for thousands of years in traditional Chinese medicine, where it's believed to have healing properties and can boost overall health. The root of this herb is used most often in cooking and teas, but you can also find ginseng supplements at many drug stores or health food stores.

Ginseng was first discovered growing wild on mountain slopes in China around 2,000 BC; since then, it has spread across Asia and North America as far north as Alaska. Today there are two main types: American ginseng (Panax quinquefolium) grows naturally in Canada and the United States--and Asian ginseng (Panax ginseng).

Aspirin or Tylenol

Aspirin, Tylenol, and other nonsteroidal anti-inflammatory drugs (NSAIDs) are often used as home remedies for relieving pain and reducing fevers. Aspirin is an acetylsalicylic acid that has been used since the 19th century to treat a variety of disorders. It is commonly taken by mouth to reduce fever, alleviate pain and treat inflammation caused by arthritis or injury.

However, these medications may have side effects such as stomach upset, bleeding ulcers, and even kidney damage if they're not taken correctly or overused in high doses. If you have been taking these medications for long periods of time or at high doses, then it's best to talk with your doctor before stopping them suddenly because this could lead to withdrawal symptoms like nausea/vomiting; dizziness/lightheadedness; headache; fatigue (feeling tired); muscle aches & pains; joint stiffness/swelling.

Echinacea

Echinacea is an herb used for centuries by Native herbs to treat colds, flu, and other ailments. It's also commonly referred to as coneflower because of its cone-shaped flower heads.

Echinacea is a perennial plant that grows in the northern hemisphere and produces purple flowers from June through September. The leaves can be dried or fresh; they have many medicinal properties, including boosting your immune system and helping with allergies!

Oregano oil

Oregano oil is a natural antibiotic that can be used to treat infections. It's also effective for sore throats, coughs, and indigestion. When taken in capsule form, it works well for colds and flu by reducing inflammation of mucus membranes in the body. The antibacterial properties of oregano make it useful for skin irritations such as acne or boils.

There are many effective natural remedies that can be used to reduce the symptoms of a cold or the flu.

When you are sick, you want to feel better as quickly as possible. Natural remedies can be effective in reducing the symptoms of a cold or the flu, and they are often healthier than over-the-counter medications. They are also affordable and easy to find at your local health food store or online.

Many herbs and essential oils help relieve congestion, reduce fever, and ease aches and pains associated with colds or flu. Some popular examples include:

The best natural herbal remedies for acne

Tea tree oil is a natural antibacterial, antifungal, and antiviral agent. It can also be used to treat mild acne by killing off the bacteria that causes it. You can use tea tree oil in many different ways:

- Dilute it with water or coconut oil and apply it directly on your face as an astringent mask. Leave for about 20 minutes before rinsing off with warm water (do not use hot water). Repeat this process once or twice a week until you see results. Apply undiluted directly onto pimples before going to bed at night -- they'll be less swollen when you wake up in the morning!

Another great ingredient for treating acne is Witch Hazel extract because of its anti-inflammatory properties, which help reduce redness and swelling associated with breakouts. Add 1 tablespoon pure witch hazel extract into 1 cup distilled witch hazel distillate (you can buy both these ingredients online). Mix well, then refrigerate until ready to use. After cleansing your face at night time, apply this mixture all over your face, including your eyelids if needed, then leave overnight before washing off in the morning with lukewarm water.

Tea Tree Oil

Tea tree oil is an effective antiseptic and can be used for skin infections, nail fungus, acne, and dandruff. It can also be used to treat warts. Tea tree oil is made from the leaves of a small evergreen shrub native to Australia called Melaleuca alternifolia, which grows in warm climates with wet winters. The oil has a distinctive odor that may be unpleasant at first but soon becomes tolerable as you use it more frequently on your skin or scalp

Witch Hazel

Witch hazel is a popular natural remedy for acne. It's an astringent that can help shrink pores and reduce inflammation.

Witch hazel can be used topically or taken internally as a toner, cleanser, or spot treatment.

Manuka Honey

Manuka honey is a type of honey that comes from bees that pollinate the Manuka bush, native to New Zealand. It's known for its antibacterial properties and has been used as an alternative medicine for centuries.

Manuka honey can be used to treat acne, wounds, and burns. It can also be used in combination with other ingredients (like tea tree oil) for different ailments like sunburns or athlete's foot.

Calendula Oil

Calendula oil is a potent natural remedy for acne. It can be applied directly to the skin or used as a carrier oil in other remedies.

Calendula oil has anti-inflammatory, antiseptic, and antibacterial properties, which make it an excellent choice for treating acne and preventing scarring caused by blemishes.

You don't need to be a scientist to use natural ingredients to treat your acne. But you do need to know how they work and how to use them safely.

- Natural ingredients can be effective but can also cause irritation and worsen your acne if you don't know what to do with them.
- How do I use natural ingredients? You can apply them directly on the skin or mix them into a solution before applying them on the face, like a toner or moisturizer (we'll get into more detail about this later).

- Are there any side effects? Some people have reported that using certain plants as topical treatments for their blemishes caused redness or itching at first, but these symptoms went away after several days of continued use--so don't give up!

Oregano Oil

Oregano oil is an essential oil that has been used for centuries as a natural remedy for various ailments. It's known for its antibacterial, antifungal, and antiviral properties.

Oregano oil can be used to treat many common illnesses like colds and flu, digestive problems such as bloating or constipation, respiratory infections like bronchitis or asthma, and fungal infections like athlete's foot or ringworm on the scalp or body (tinea versicolor). The active ingredient in oregano oil is carvacrol which is responsible for these beneficial effects.

These herbs can be used for many different ailments.

- These herbs can be used for many different ailments.
- They are also good for your immune system.
- They can help you prevent illness, manage pain and boost your immune system.

Some of the herbs that you can use are:

These herbs are great for managing pain, boosting your immune system, and preventing illness. They're also affordable and easy to find at most health stores or online retailers. So, if you're looking for a natural remedy that works well with your body instead of against it, try some herbal remedies today!

Chapter 06 Herbal Recipes

Herbal Teas Recipes

Chamomile Tea

Ingredients:

1 tablespoon dried chamomile flowers

1 cup boiling water

Optional: honey or lemon to taste

Instructions:

Place the dried chamomile flowers in a tea infuser or tea bag.

Pour boiling water over the tea infuser or tea bag.

Steep for 5-10 minutes.

Remove the tea infuser or tea bag and add honey or lemon to taste, if desired.

Preparation Time: 5-10 minutes

Servings: 1

Peppermint Tea

Ingredients:

1 tablespoon dried peppermint leaves   Optional: honey to taste

1 cup boiling water

Instructions:

Place the dried peppermint leaves in a tea infuser or tea bag.

Pour boiling water over the tea infuser or tea bag.

Steep for 5-10 minutes.

Remove the tea infuser or tea bag and add honey to taste, if desired.

Preparation Time: 5-10 minutes

Servings: 1

Lemon Balm Tea

Ingredients:

1 tablespoon dried lemon balm leaves

1 cup boiling water

Optional: honey to taste

Instructions:

Place the dried lemon balm leaves in a tea infuser or tea bag.

Pour boiling water over the tea infuser or tea bag.

Steep for 5-10 minutes.

Remove the tea infuser or tea bag and add honey to taste, if desired.

Preparation Time: 5-10 minutes

Servings: 1

Lavender Tea

Ingredients:

1 tablespoon dried lavender flowers

1 cup boiling water

Optional: honey to taste

Instructions:

Place the dried lavender flowers in a tea infuser or tea bag.

Pour boiling water over the tea infuser or tea bag.

Steep for 5-10 minutes.

Remove the tea infuser or tea bag and add honey to taste, if desired.

Preparation Time: 5-10 minutes

Servings: 1

Ginger Tea

Ingredients:

1 tablespoon grated fresh ginger root

1 cup boiling water

Optional: honey or lemon to taste

Instructions:

Place the grated ginger root in a tea infuser or tea bag.

Pour boiling water over the tea infuser or tea bag.

Steep for 5-10 minutes.

Remove the tea infuser or tea bag and add honey or lemon to taste, if desired.

Preparation Time: 5-10 minutes

Servings: 1

Hibiscus Tea

Ingredients:

1 tablespoon dried hibiscus flowers

1 cup boiling water

Optional: honey or lemon to taste

Instructions:

Place the dried hibiscus flowers in a tea infuser or tea bag.

Pour boiling water over the tea infuser or tea bag.

Steep for 5-10 minutes.

Remove the tea infuser or tea bag and add honey or lemon to taste, if desired.

Preparation Time: 5-10 minutes

Servings: 1

Cinnamon Tea

Ingredients:

1 cinnamon stick or 1 teaspoon ground cinnamon

1 cup boiling water

Optional: honey to taste

Instructions:

Place the cinnamon stick or ground cinnamon in a tea infuser or tea bag.

Pour boiling water over the tea infuser or tea bag.

Steep for 5-10 minutes.

Remove the tea infuser or tea bag and add honey to taste, if desired.

Preparation Time: 5-10 minutes

Servings: 1

Nettle Tea

Ingredients:

1 tablespoon dried nettle leaves

Optional: honey or lemon to taste

1 cup boiling water

Instructions:

Place the dried nettle leaves in a tea infuser or tea bag.

Pour boiling water over the tea infuser or tea bag.

Steep for 5-10 minutes.

Remove the tea infuser or tea bag and add honey or lemon to taste, if desired.

Preparation Time: 5-10 minutes

Servings: 1

Fennel Tea

Ingredients:

1 tablespoon fennel seeds

Optional: honey to taste

1 cup boiling water

Instructions:

Place the fennel seeds in a tea infuser or tea bag.

Pour boiling water over the tea infuser or tea bag.

Steep for 5-10 minutes.

Remove the tea infuser or tea bag and add honey to taste, if desired.

Preparation Time: 5-10 minutes

Servings: 1

Lemon Ginger Tea

Ingredients:

1 tablespoon grated fresh ginger root

1 tablespoon fresh lemon juice

1 cup boiling water

Optional: honey to taste

Instructions:

Place the grated ginger root in a tea infuser or tea bag.

Pour boiling water over the tea infuser or tea bag.

Add fresh lemon juice to the tea.

Steep for 5-10 minutes.

Remove the tea infuser or tea bag and add honey to taste, if desired.

Preparation Time: 5-10 minutes

Servings: 1

Rose Tea

Ingredients:

1 tablespoon dried rose petals

1 cup boiling water

Optional: honey or milk to taste

Instructions:

Place the dried rose petals in a tea infuser or tea bag.

Pour boiling water over the tea infuser or tea bag.

Steep for 5-10 minutes.

Remove the tea infuser or tea bag and add honey or milk to taste, if desired.

Preparation Time: 5-10 minutes

Servings: 1

Mentha piperita Tea

Ingredients:

1 tablespoon dried peppermint leaves

Optional: honey to taste

1 cup boiling water

Instructions:

Place the dried peppermint leaves in a tea infuser or tea bag.

Pour boiling water over the tea infuser or tea bag.

Steep for 5-10 minutes.

Remove the tea infuser or tea bag and add honey to taste, if desired.

Preparation Time: 5-10 minutes

Servings: 1

Chamomile Tea

Ingredients:

1 tablespoon dried chamomile flowers

Optional: honey to taste

1 cup boiling water

Instructions:

Place the dried chamomile flowers in a tea infuser or tea bag.

Pour boiling water over the tea infuser or tea bag.

Steep for 5-10 minutes.

Remove the tea infuser or tea bag and add honey to taste, if desired.

Preparation Time: 5-10 minutes

Servings: 1

Turmeric Tea

Ingredients:

1 teaspoon ground turmeric

1 teaspoon grated fresh ginger root

1 tablespoon honey

1 tablespoon lemon juice

Instructions:

Place the ground turmeric and grated ginger root in a tea infuser or tea bag.

Pour boiling water over the tea infuser or tea bag.

Add honey and lemon juice to the tea.

Servings: 1

Lemon Balm Tea

Ingredients:

1 tablespoon dried lemon balm leaves

1 cup boiling water

Instructions:

Place the dried lemon balm leaves in a tea infuser or tea bag.

Pour boiling water over the tea infuser or tea bag.

Steep for 5-10 minutes.

Remove the tea infuser or tea bag and add honey to taste, if desired.

Preparation Time: 5-10 minutes

Servings: 1

1 cup boiling water

Steep for 5-10 minutes.

Remove the tea infuser or tea bag and serve.

Preparation Time: 5-10 minutes

Optional: honey to taste

Infused Oils Recipes

Garlic-Infused Olive Oil

Ingredients:

1 cup extra-virgin olive oil

2-3 cloves garlic

Instructions:

Peel the garlic cloves and slice them thinly.

Add the sliced garlic to a clean, dry glass jar.

Pour the olive oil over the garlic, making sure the garlic is completely covered.

Cover the jar with a lid and store it in a cool, dark place for at least a week.

Strain the oil through a fine mesh strainer or cheesecloth to remove the garlic.

Preparation Time: 10 minutes

Servings: Approximately 1 cup

Rosemary-Infused Olive Oil

Ingredients:

1 cup extra-virgin olive oil

1/4 cup fresh rosemary leaves

Instructions:

Wash and dry the rosemary leaves.

Add the rosemary leaves to a clean, dry glass jar.

Pour the olive oil over the rosemary leaves, making sure the leaves are completely covered.

Cover the jar with a lid and store it in a cool, dark place for at least a week.

Strain the oil through a fine mesh strainer or cheesecloth to remove the rosemary leaves.

Preparation Time: 10 minutes

Servings: Approximately 1 cup

Lemon-Infused Olive Oil

Ingredients:

1 cup extra-virgin olive oil

1-2 lemons

Instructions:

Wash and dry the lemons.

Use a vegetable peeler to remove the zest from the lemons in long, thin strips.

Add the lemon zest to a clean, dry glass jar.

Pour the olive oil over the lemon zest, making sure the zest is completely covered.

Cover the jar with a lid and store it in a cool, dark place for at least a week.

Strain the oil through a fine mesh strainer or cheesecloth to remove the lemon zest.

Preparation Time: 10 minutes

Servings: Approximately 1 cup

Basil-Infused Olive Oil

Ingredients:

1 cup extra-virgin olive oil

1/2 cup fresh basil leaves

Instructions:

Wash and dry the basil leaves.

Add the basil leaves to a clean, dry glass jar.

Pour the olive oil over the basil leaves, making sure the leaves are completely covered.

Cover the jar with a lid and store it in a cool, dark place for at least a week.

Strain the oil through a fine mesh strainer or cheesecloth to remove the basil leaves.

Preparation Time: 10 minutes

Servings: Approximately 1 cup

Chili-Infused Olive Oil

Ingredients:

1 cup extra-virgin olive oil

2-3 dried chili peppers

Instructions:

Remove the stems from the chili peppers

Add the chili peppers to a clean, dry glass jar.

Pour the olive oil over the chili peppers, making sure the peppers are completely covered.

Cover the jar with a lid and store it in a cool, dark place for at least a week.

Strain the oil through a fine mesh strainer or cheesecloth to remove the chili peppers.

Preparation Time: 10 minutes

Servings: Approximately 1 cup

Thyme-Infused Olive Oil

Ingredients:

1 cup extra-virgin olive oil   1/2 cup fresh thyme leaves

Instructions:

Wash and dry the thyme leaves.

Add the thyme leaves to a clean, dry glass jar.

Pour the olive oil over the thyme leaves, making sure the leaves are completely covered.

Cover the jar with a lid and store it in a cool, dark place for at least a week.

Strain the oil through a fine mesh strainer or cheesecloth to remove the thyme leaves.

Preparation Time: 10 minutes

Servings: Approximately 1 cup

Cinnamon-Infused Olive Oil

Ingredients:

1 cup extra-virgin olive oil   3 cinnamon sticks

Instructions:

Break the cinnamon sticks into small pieces.

Add the cinnamon pieces to a clean, dry glass jar.

Pour the olive oil over the cinnamon pieces, making sure the pieces are completely covered.

Cover the jar with a lid and store it in a cool, dark place for at least a week.

Strain the oil through a fine mesh strainer or cheesecloth to remove the cinnamon pieces.

Preparation Time: 10 minutes

Servings: Approximately 1 cup

Lavender-Infused Olive Oil

Ingredients:

1 cup extra-virgin olive oil   1/2 cup fresh lavender flowers

Instructions:

Wash and dry the lavender flowers.

Add the lavender flowers to a clean, dry glass jar.

Pour the olive oil over the lavender flowers, making sure the flowers are completely covered.

Cover the jar with a lid and store it in a cool, dark place for at least a week.

Strain the oil through a fine mesh strainer or cheesecloth to remove the lavender flowers.

Preparation Time: 10 minutes

Servings: Approximately 1 cup

Sage-Infused Olive Oil

Ingredients:

1 cup extra-virgin olive oil   1/2 cup fresh sage leaves

Instructions:

Wash and dry the sage leaves.

Add the sage leaves to a clean, dry glass jar.

Pour the olive oil over the sage leaves, making sure the leaves are completely covered.

Cover the jar with a lid and store it in a cool, dark place for at least a week.

Strain the oil through a fine mesh strainer or cheesecloth to remove the sage leaves.

Preparation Time: 10 minutes

Servings: Approximately 1 cup

Garlic-Infused Olive Oil

Ingredients:

1 cup extra-virgin olive oil   4-5 garlic cloves, sliced

Instructions:

Peel and slice the garlic cloves.

Add the sliced garlic to a clean, dry glass jar.

Pour the olive oil over the garlic, making sure the garlic is completely covered.

Cover the jar with a lid and store it in a cool, dark place for at least a week.

Strain the oil through a fine mesh strainer or cheesecloth to remove the garlic.

Preparation Time: 10 minutes

Servings: Approximately 1 cup

Rosemary-Infused Olive Oil

Ingredients:

1 cup extra-virgin olive oil   1/2 cup fresh rosemary leaves

Instructions:

Wash and dry the rosemary leaves.

Add the rosemary leaves to a clean, dry glass jar.

Pour the olive oil over the rosemary leaves, making sure the leaves are completely covered.

Cover the jar with a lid and store it in a cool, dark place for at least a week.

Strain the oil through a fine mesh strainer or cheesecloth to remove the rosemary leaves.

Preparation Time: 10 minutes

Servings: Approximately 1 cup

Lemon-Infused Olive Oil

Ingredients:

1 cup extra-virgin olive oil   1-2 lemons, thinly sliced

Instructions:

Wash and thinly slice the lemons.

Add the sliced lemons to a clean, dry glass jar.

Pour the olive oil over the lemons, making sure the lemons are completely covered.

Cover the jar with a lid and store it in a cool, dark place for at least a week.

Strain the oil through a fine mesh strainer or cheesecloth to remove the lemon slices.

Preparation Time: 10 minutes

Servings: Approximately 1 cup

Herbal Tinctures Recipes

Echinacea Tincture

Ingredients:

1 cup dried echinacea root

2 cups 80-proof alcohol (such as vodka or brandy)

Instructions:

Finely chop or grind the dried echinacea root.

Add the echinacea root to a clean, dry glass jar.

Pour the alcohol over the echinacea root, making sure it's completely covered.

Stir or shake the mixture to combine.

Store the jar in a cool, dark place for 4-6 weeks, shaking it daily.

Strain the tincture through a cheesecloth or fine mesh strainer.

Transfer the tincture to a dark glass dropper bottle and label it.

Preparation Time: 10 minutes

Servings: Approximately 48 (based on a 30-drop serving size)

Valerian Root Tincture

Ingredients:

1 cup dried valerian root

2 cups 80-proof alcohol (such as vodka or brandy)

Instructions:

Finely chop or grind the dried valerian root.

Add the valerian root to a clean, dry glass jar.

Pour the alcohol over the valerian root, making sure it's completely covered.

Stir or shake the mixture to combine.

Store the jar in a cool, dark place for 4-6 weeks, shaking it daily.

Strain the tincture through a cheesecloth or fine mesh strainer.

Transfer the tincture to a dark glass dropper bottle and label it.

Preparation Time: 10 minutes

Servings: Approximately 48 (based on a 30-drop serving size)

Milk Thistle Tincture

Ingredients:

1 cup dried milk thistle seeds

2 cups 80-proof alcohol (such as vodka or brandy)

Instructions:

Finely chop or grind the dried milk thistle seeds.

Add the milk thistle seeds to a clean, dry glass jar.

Pour the alcohol over the milk thistle seeds, making sure it's completely covered.

Stir or shake the mixture to combine.

Store the jar in a cool, dark place for 4-6 weeks, shaking it daily.

Strain the tincture through a cheesecloth or fine mesh strainer.

Transfer the tincture to a dark glass dropper bottle and label it.

Preparation Time: 10 minutes

Servings: Approximately 48 (based on a 30-drop serving size)

Ginger Tincture

Ingredients:

1 cup fresh ginger root, chopped

2 cups 80-proof alcohol (such as vodka or brandy)

Instructions:

Wash and chop the fresh ginger root.

Add the chopped ginger to a clean, dry glass jar.

Pour the alcohol over the ginger, making sure it's completely covered.

Stir or shake the mixture to combine.

Store the jar in a cool, dark place for 4-6 weeks, shaking it daily.

6. Strain the tincture through a cheesecloth or fine mesh strainer.

Transfer the tincture to a dark glass dropper bottle and label it.

Preparation Time: 10 minutes

Servings: Approximately 48 (based on a 30-drop serving size)

Passionflower Tincture

Ingredients:

1 cup dried passionflower

2 cups 80-proof alcohol (such as vodka or brandy)

Instructions:

Finely chop or grind the dried passionflower.

Add the passionflower to a clean, dry glass jar.

Pour the alcohol over the passionflower, making sure it's completely covered.

Stir or shake the mixture to combine.

Store the jar in a cool, dark place for 4-6 weeks, shaking it daily.

Strain the tincture through a cheesecloth or fine mesh strainer.

Transfer the tincture to a dark glass dropper bottle and label it.

Preparation Time: 10 minutes

Servings: Approximately 48 (based on a 30-drop serving size)

Dandelion Root Tincture

Ingredients:

1 cup dried dandelion root

2 cups 80-proof alcohol (such as vodka or brandy)

Instructions:

Finely chop or grind the dried dandelion root.

Add the dandelion root to a clean, dry glass jar.

Pour the alcohol over the dandelion root, making sure it's completely covered.

Stir or shake the mixture to combine.

Store the jar in a cool, dark place for 4-6 weeks, shaking it daily.

Strain the tincture through a cheesecloth or fine mesh strainer.

Transfer the tincture to a dark glass dropper bottle and label it.

Preparation Time: 10 minutes

Servings: Approximately 48 (based on a 30-drop serving size)

Hawthorn Berry Tincture

Ingredients:

1 cup dried hawthorn berries

2 cups 80-proof alcohol (such as vodka or brandy)

Instructions:

Finely chop or grind the dried hawthorn berries.

Add the hawthorn berries to a clean, dry glass jar.

Pour the alcohol over the hawthorn berries, making sure it's completely covered.

Stir or shake the mixture to combine.

Store the jar in a cool, dark place for 4-6 weeks, shaking it daily.

Strain the tincture through a cheesecloth or fine mesh strainer.

Transfer the tincture to a dark glass dropper bottle and label it.

Preparation Time: 10 minutes

Servings: Approximately 48 (based on a 30-drop serving size)

Astragalus Tincture

Ingredients:

1 cup dried aster alalus root

2 cups 80-proof alcohol (such as vodka or brandy)

Instructions:

Finely chop or grind the dried astragalus root.

Add the astragalus root to a clean, dry glass jar.

Pour the alcohol over the astragalus root, making sure it's completely covered.

Stir or shake the mixture to combine.

Store the jar in a cool, dark place for 4-6 weeks, shaking it daily.

Strain the tincture through a cheesecloth or fine mesh strainer.

Transfer the tincture to a dark glass dropper bottle and label it.

Preparation Time: 10 minutes

Servings: Approximately 48 (based on a 30-drop serving size)

Exploit Thistle Tincture

Ingredients:

1 cup dried milk thistle seeds

2 cups 80-proof alcohol (such as vodka or brandy)

Instructions:

Finely chop or grind the dried milk thistle seeds.

Add the milk thistle seeds to a clean, dry glass jar.

Pour the alcohol over the milk thistle seeds, making sure it's completely covered.

Stir or shake the mixture to combine.

Store the jar in a cool, dark place for 4-6 weeks, shaking it daily.

Strain the tincture through a cheesecloth or fine mesh strainer.

Transfer the tincture to a dark glass dropper bottle and label it.

Preparation Time: 10 minutes

Servings: Approximately 48 (based on a 30-drop serving size)

Lemon Balm Tincture

Ingredients:

1 cup dried lemon balm

2 cups 80-proof alcohol (such as vodka or brandy)

Instructions:

Finely chop or grind the dried lemon balm.

Add the lemon balm to a clean, dry glass jar.

Pour the alcohol over the lemon balm, making sure it's completely covered.

Stir or shake the mixture to combine.

Store the jar in a cool, dark place for 4-6 weeks, shaking it daily.

Strain the tincture through a cheesecloth or fine mesh strainer.

Transfer the tincture to a dark glass dropper bottle and label it.

Preparation Time: 10 minutes

Servings: Approximately 48 (based on a 30-drop serving size)

Herbal Culinary Recipes

Rosemary Roasted Potatoes

Ingredients:

2 lbs. baby potatoes, halved

3 tbsp olive oil

2 tbsp fresh rosemary, chopped

Salt and pepper to taste

Instructions:

Preheat the oven to 400°F.

Toss the potatoes with the olive oil, rosemary, salt, and pepper.

Spread the potatoes out in a single layer on a baking sheet.

Roast the potatoes for 25-30 minutes or until they are golden brown and crispy.

Preparation Time: 35 minutes

Servings: 6

Basil Pesto

Ingredients:

2 cups fresh basil leaves

1/2 cup grated Parmesan cheese

1/2 cup extra-virgin olive oil

1/3 cup pine nuts

3 garlic cloves, peeled

Salt and pepper to taste

Instructions:

In a food processor, combine the basil, Parmesan, olive oil, pine nuts, garlic, salt, and pepper.

Process until smooth and well combined.

Taste and adjust the seasoning as needed.

Preparation Time: 10 minutes

Servings: 8

Lavender Lemonade

Ingredients:

1 cup fresh squeezed lemon juice

1/2 cup honey

8 cups water

1/4 cup fresh lavender buds

Instructions:

In a small saucepan, bring the honey, lavender buds, and 2 cups of water to a boil.

Reduce the heat and simmer for 5 minutes.

Remove from heat and let cool for 10 minutes.

Strain out the lavender buds.

Servings: 8

In a large pitcher, combine the lemon juice, lavender honey mixture, and remaining water.

Stir well and refrigerate until cold.

Preparation Time: 20 minutes

Chive Butter

Ingredients:

1/2 cup unsalted butter, softened

2 tbsp fresh chives, chopped

Salt and pepper to taste

Instructions:

In a small bowl, combine the butter, chives, salt, and pepper.

Mix well until the ingredients are evenly distributed.

Transfer the butter to a small serving dish and refrigerate until ready to use.

Preparation Time: 5 minutes

Servings: 8

Sage and Mushroom Risotto

Ingredients:

6 cups chicken or vegetable broth

2 tbsp olive oil

1 onion, diced

2 cloves garlic, minced

1 lb. mushrooms, sliced

1 1/2 cups Arborio rice

1/2 cup white wine

1/4 cup fresh sage leaves, chopped

1/2 cup grated Parmesan cheese

Salt and pepper to taste

Instructions:

In a medium saucepan, bring the broth to a simmer.

In a large, heavy-bottomed pot, heat the olive oil over medium heat.

Add the onion and garlic and cook until the onion is translucent.

Add the mushrooms and cook until they release their moisture and become tender.

Add the rice to the pot and stir to coat it in the oil.

Add the white wine and stir until it is absorbed.

Add a ladleful of the simmering broth to the pot and stir until it is absorbed.

Repeat, adding one ladleful of broth at a time and stirring until it is absorbed until the rice is tender and the mixture is creamy.

Stir in the chopped sage and Parmesan cheese.

Preparation Time: 45 minutes

Servings: 6

Mint Yogurt Sauce

Ingredients:

1 cup plain Greek yogurt

1/4 cup fresh mint leaves, chopped

1 clove garlic, minced

1 tbsp lemon juice

Salt and pepper to taste

Instructions:

In a small bowl, combine the yogurt, mint, garlic, lemon juice, salt, and pepper.

Mix well until the ingredients are evenly distributed.

Cover and refrigerate until ready to use.

Preparation Time: 5 minutes

Servings: 4

Thyme and Garlic Roasted Chicken

Ingredients:

1 whole chicken, about 4 lbs.

2 tbsp olive oil

2 tbsp fresh thyme leaves

4 cloves garlic, minced

Salt and pepper to taste

Instructions:

Preheat the oven to 425°F.

In a small bowl, combine the olive oil, thyme, garlic, salt, and pepper.

Rub the mixture all over the chicken, making sure to coat it evenly.

Place the chicken in a roasting pan and roast for 50-60 minutes or until the internal temperature reaches 165°F.

Let the chicken rest for 10-15 minutes before carving.

Preparation Time: 1 hour and 15 minutes

Servings: 6

Dill Potato Salad

Ingredients:

2 lbs. baby potatoes, boiled and chopped

1/2 cup mayonnaise

1/4 cup plain Greek yogurt

2 tbsp fresh dill, chopped

2 tbsp Dijon mustard

2 cloves garlic, minced

Salt and pepper to taste

Instructions:

In a large bowl, combine the mayonnaise, yogurt, dill, mustard, garlic, salt, and pepper.

Add the chopped potatoes and stir until they are coated in the dressing.

Cover and refrigerate for at least 1 hour before serving.

Preparation Time: 1 hour and 15 minutes

Servings: 6

Parsley and Lemon Quinoa

Ingredients:

1 cup quinoa, rinsed

2 cups water

1/4 cup fresh parsley, chopped

1 clove garlic, minced

2 tbsp lemon juice

2 tbsp olive oil

Salt and pepper to taste

Instructions:

In a medium saucepan, combine the quinoa and water.

Bring to a boil over high heat.

Reduce the heat to low and cover.

Simmer for 15-20 minutes or until the quinoa is tender and the water is absorbed.

In a small bowl, whisk together the parsley, garlic, lemon juice, olive oil, salt, and pepper.

Fluff the quinoa with a fork and stir in the parsley mixture.

Serve warm or chilled.

Preparation Time: 25 minutes

Servings: 4

Sage and Thyme Pork Chops

Ingredients:

4 pork chops, about 1 inch thick

2 tbsp olive oil

2 tbsp fresh sage, chopped

2 tbsp fresh thyme, chopped

2 cloves garlic, minced

Salt and pepper to taste

Instructions:

Preheat the oven to 375°F.

In a small bowl, combine the olive oil, sage, thyme, garlic, salt, and pepper.

Rub the mixture all over the pork chops, making sure to coat them evenly.

Heat a large, oven-safe skillet over medium-high heat.

Add the pork chops to the skillet and cook for 3-4 minutes on each side or until browned.

Transfer the skillet to the oven and bake for 10-15 minutes or until the internal temperature reaches 145°F.

Let the pork chops rest for 5 minutes before serving.

Preparation Time: 30 minutes

Servings: 4

Basil Pesto Pasta

Ingredients:

12 oz linguine

2 cups fresh basil leaves, packed

1/2 cup grated Parmesan cheese

1/4 cup pine nuts

2 cloves garlic, minced

1/2 cup olive oil

Salt and pepper to taste

Instructions:

Cook the linguine according to the package instructions.

While the pasta cooks, combine the basil, Parmesan, pine nuts, garlic, salt, and pepper in a food processor.

Pulse until the ingredients are finely chopped.

With the food processor running, slowly pour in the olive oil until the mixture is smooth and creamy.

Drain the pasta and return it to the pot.

Add the pesto sauce and toss to coat the pasta evenly.

Serve immediately.

Preparation Time: 1 hour and 15 minutes

Servings: 6

Lavender Lemon Bars

Ingredients:

1 1/2 cups all-purpose flour	1 1/2 cups granulated sugar
1/2 cup powdered sugar	1/4 cup fresh lemon juice
3/4 cup unsalted butter, softened	1 tbsp lemon zest
4 eggs	1 tbsp dried lavender buds

Instructions:

Preheat the oven to 350°F.

In a medium bowl, combine the flour, powdered sugar, and 1/4 cup of the granulated sugar.

Cut in the butter until the mixture resembles coarse crumbs.

Press the mixture into the bottom of a 9x13-inch baking dish.

Bake for 15-20 minutes or until lightly golden.

While the crust bakes, whisk together the eggs, remaining 1 1/4 cups of granulated sugar, lemon juice, lemon zest, and lavender buds in a medium bowl.

Pour the mixture over the baked crust.

Bake for an additional 25-30 minutes or until the filling is set and lightly golden.

Let the bars cool completely before slicing and serving.

Preparation Time: 1 hour and 15 minutes

Servings: 12

Rosemary Roasted Potatoes
Ingredients:

2 lbs. small red potatoes, quartered

2 tbsp olive oil

2 tbsp fresh rosemary, chopped

Salt and pepper to taste

Instructions:

Preheat the oven to 400°F.

In a large bowl, toss the potatoes with the olive oil, rosemary, salt, and pepper.

Spread the potatoes out on a baking sheet in a single layer.

Bake for 30-35 minutes or until the potatoes are tender and golden brown.

Serve immediately.

Preparation Time: 45 minutes

Servings: 4

Mint Chocolate Chip Ice Cream

Ingredients:

2 cups heavy cream

1 cup whole milk

3/4 cup granulated sugar

2 tbsp fresh mint leaves, chopped

5 egg yolks

1/2 tsp vanilla extract

1/2 cup semisweet chocolate chips

Instructions:

In a medium saucepan, heat the cream, milk, sugar, and mint leaves over medium heat until the mixture is hot and steamy but not boiling.

In a separate bowl, whisk the egg yolks until they are pale and frothy.

Slowly pour the hot cream mixture into the egg yolks, whisking constantly.

Pour the mixture back into the saucepan and heat over medium-low heat, stirring constantly, until it thickens and coats the back of a spoon.

Remove from heat and stir in the vanilla extract.

Strain the mixture through a fine mesh sieve to remove the mint leaves.

Chill the mixture in the refrigerator for at least 2 hours or until completely cooled.

Churn the mixture in an ice cream maker according to the manufacturer's instructions.

During the last few minutes of churning, add the chocolate chips.

Transfer the ice cream to a freezer-safe container and freeze for at least 2 hours or until firm.

Serve and enjoy.

Preparation Time: 3 hours and 30 minutes

Servings: 6

Sage and Brown Butter Pasta

Ingredients:

12 oz linguine

1/2 cup unsalted butter

1/4 cup fresh sage leaves

1/2 cup grated Parmesan cheese

Salt and pepper to taste

Instructions:

Cook the linguine according to the package instructions.

While the pasta cooks, melt the butter in a large skillet over medium heat.

Cook the butter until it turns golden brown and smells nutty, stirring occasionally.

Add the sage leaves and cook for 1-2 minutes or until crispy.

Drain the pasta and add it to the skillet with the brown butter and sage.

Toss to coat the pasta evenly.

Add the Parmesan cheese, salt, and pepper, and toss again.

Serve immediately.

Preparation Time: 30 minutes

Servings: 4

Herbal Condiments Recipes

Garlic and Herb Butter

Ingredients:

1 stick unsalted butter, room temperature

2 cloves garlic, minced

1 tablespoon chopped fresh parsley

1 teaspoon chopped fresh thyme

1 teaspoon chopped fresh rosemary

Instructions:

In a mixing bowl, combine the butter, garlic, parsley, thyme, and rosemary until well mixed.

Transfer the mixture to a small bowl and cover with plastic wrap.

Refrigerate for at least 30 minutes or until ready to use.

Preparation time: 10 minutes

Servings: 8

Italian Herb Seasoning

Ingredients:

1 tablespoon dried basil

1 tablespoon dried oregano

1 tablespoon dried thyme

1 tablespoon dried rosemary

1 tablespoon garlic powder

1 tablespoon onion powder

1 teaspoon sea salt

Instructions:

In a small bowl, combine all ingredients and mix well.

Store in an airtight container until ready to use.

Preparation time: 5 minutes

Servings: 8

Chimichurri Sauce

Ingredients:

1/2 cup fresh parsley, chopped

1/4 cup fresh oregano, chopped

1/4 cup fresh cilantro, chopped

2 garlic cloves, minced

1/2 cup olive oil

2 tablespoons red wine vinegar

1 teaspoon sea salt

1/4 teaspoon red pepper flakes

Instructions:

In a mixing bowl, combine all ingredients and mix well.

Store in an airtight container in the refrigerator for up to one week.

Preparation time: 10 minutes

Servings: 8

Lemon Dill Yogurt Sauce

Ingredients:

1 cup plain Greek yogurt

1 tablespoon chopped fresh dill

1 teaspoon lemon zest

1 tablespoon fresh lemon juice

1 garlic clove, minced

1/4 teaspoon sea salt

Instructions:

In a mixing bowl, combine all ingredients and mix well.

Store in an airtight container in the refrigerator for up to one week.

Preparation time: 5 minutes

Servings: 6

Herbs de Provence

Ingredients:

2 tablespoons dried thyme

2 tablespoons dried rosemary

2 tablespoons dried oregano

2 tablespoons dried marjoram

2 tablespoons dried savory

Instructions:

In a small bowl, combine all ingredients and mix well.

Store in an airtight container until ready to use.

Preparation time: 5 minutes

Servings: 8

Basil Pesto:
Ingredients:

2 cups fresh basil leaves

2 garlic cloves, minced

1/2 cup grated Parmesan cheese

1/2 cup olive oil

1/2 cup pine nuts

1/4 teaspoon sea salt

Instructions:

In a food processor, combine the basil, Parmesan cheese, pine nuts, garlic, and salt.

Pulse until finely chopped.

While the processor is running, slowly drizzle in the olive oil until the pesto is smooth.

Store in an airtight container in the refrigerator for up to one week.

Preparation time: 15 minutes

Servings: 8

Spicy Mustard
Ingredients:

1/2 cup yellow mustard seeds

1 teaspoon honey

1/2 cup apple cider vinegar

1/4 teaspoon sea salt

1/4 cup water

1/4 teaspoon cayenne pepper

Instructions:

In a mixing bowl, combine the mustard seeds, apple cider vinegar, and water.

Cover with plastic wrap and let soak at room temperature for 24 hours.

Transfer the mixture to a food processor and add the honey, salt, and cayenne pepper.

Process until smooth.

Store in an airtight container in the refrigerator for up to one month.

Preparation time: 5 minutes plus 24 hours for soaking

Servings: 8

Cilantro Lime Dressing

Ingredients:

1/2 cup chopped fresh cilantro

1/4 cup olive oil

1/4 teaspoon sea salt

1/4 cup fresh lime juice

1 garlic clove, minced

Instructions:

In a mixing bowl, combine all ingredients and mix well.

Store in an airtight container in the refrigerator for up to one week.

Preparation time: 5 minutes

Servings: 6

Rosemary Infused Olive Oil

Ingredients:

1 cup extra-virgin olive oil

2 sprigs of fresh rosemary

Instructions:

In a small saucepan, heat the olive oil and rosemary over low heat.

Heat for 10-15 minutes or until the rosemary becomes fragrant.

Remove from heat and let cool.

Strain the oil and discard the rosemary.

Store in an airtight container in a cool, dark place for up to one month.

Preparation time: 15 minutes

Servings: 8

Curry Powder

Ingredients:

1 tablespoon ground cumin

1 tablespoon ground coriander

1 tablespoon ground turmeric

1 teaspoon ground ginger

1/2 teaspoon ground cinnamon

1/2 teaspoon cayenne pepper

Instructions:

In a small bowl, combine all ingredients and mix well.

Store in an airtight container until ready to use.

Preparation time: 5 minutes

Servings: 8

Tarragon Mustard

Ingredients:

1/2 cup Dijon mustard

2 tablespoons chopped fresh tarragon

1 tablespoon honey

Instructions:

In a mixing bowl, combine all ingredients and mix well.

Store in an airtight container in the refrigerator for up to one month.

Preparation time: 5 minutes

Servings: 8

Tomato and Basil Salsa

Ingredients:

2 cups chopped fresh tomatoes

1/4 cup chopped fresh basil

1 garlic clove, minced

1 tablespoon olive oil

1 tablespoon balsamic vinegar

1/4 teaspoon sea salt

Instructions:

In a mixing bowl, combine all ingredients and mix well.

Store in an airtight container in the refrigerator for up to one week.

Preparation time: 10 minutes

Servings: 6

Recipes for Herbal Cocktails and Mocktails

Lavender Lemonade Cocktail

Ingredients: 2 oz vodka, 2 oz fresh lemon juice, 1 oz lavender simple syrup, 4 oz sparkling water, lavender sprigs for garnish

Instructions: In a shaker, combine vodka, lemon juice, and lavender syrup with ice. Shake until well combined. Strain into a glass filled with ice. Top with sparkling water and garnish with lavender sprigs.

Preparation time: 5 minutes

Servings: 1

Rosemary Gin and Tonic

Ingredients: 2 oz gin, 4 oz tonic water, 1 sprig of fresh rosemary, lime wedge for garnish

Instructions: In a glass, muddle the rosemary sprig. Add ice, gin, and tonic water. Stir gently. Squeeze the lime wedge into the glass and garnish with a sprig of rosemary.

Preparation time: 5 minutes

Servings: 1

Hibiscus Margarita

Ingredients: 2 oz tequila, 1 oz hibiscus syrup, 1 oz fresh lime juice, 1/2 oz triple sec, hibiscus flowers for garnish

Instructions: In a shaker, combine tequila, hibiscus syrup, lime juice, and triple sec with ice. Shake until well combined. Strain into a glass filled with ice. Garnish with hibiscus flowers.

Preparation time: 5 minutes

Servings: 1

Mint Mojito Mocktail

Ingredients: 1/2 cup fresh mint leaves, 1 oz lime juice, 1 oz simple syrup, 4 oz sparkling water, lime wedges and mint sprigs for garnish

Instructions: In a glass, muddle the mint leaves. Add ice, lime juice, and simple syrup. Stir gently. Top with sparkling water. Garnish with lime wedges and mint sprigs.

Preparation time: 5 minutes

Servings: 1

Thyme and Grapefruit Vodka Spritzer

Ingredients: 2 oz vodka, 1 oz thyme simple syrup, 2 oz fresh grapefruit juice, 2 oz sparkling water, grapefruit wedges and thyme sprigs for garnish

Instructions: In a shaker, combine vodka, thyme syrup, and grapefruit juice with ice. Shake until well combined. Strain into a glass filled with ice. Top with sparkling water. Garnish with grapefruit wedges and thyme sprigs.

Preparation time: 5 minutes

Servings: 1

Sage and Blackberry Gin Fizz

Ingredients: 2 oz gin, 1 oz blackberry simple syrup, 1 oz fresh lime juice, 2 oz club soda, fresh sage leaves and blackberries for garnish

Instructions: In a shaker, combine gin, blackberry syrup, and lime juice with ice. Shake until well combined. Strain into a glass filled with ice. Top with club soda. Garnish with fresh sage leaves and blackberries.

Preparation time: 5 minutes

Servings: 1

Cucumber and Basil Gin and Tonic

Ingredients: 2 oz gin, 4 oz tonic water, 2 cucumber slices, 2 fresh basil leaves, lime wedge for garnish

Instructions: In a glass, muddle the cucumber slices and basil leaves. Add ice, gin, and tonic water. Stir gently. Squeeze the lime wedge into the glass and garnish with a cucumber slice.

Preparation time: 5 minutes

Servings: 1

Chamomile and Honey Whiskey Sour

Ingredients: 2 oz whiskey, 1 oz chamomile tea, 1/2 oz honey, 1 oz fresh lemon juice, lemon slice and chamomile flowers for garnish

Instructions: In a shaker, combine whiskey, chamomile tea, honey, and lemon juice with ice. Shake until well combined. Strain into a glass filled with ice. Garnish with a lemon slice and chamomile flowers.

Preparation time: 5 minutes

Servings: 1

Ginger and Lemongrass Sparkling Water

Ingredients: 1 cup sparkling water, 1-inch piece of fresh ginger, 1 stalk of fresh lemongrass, a lime wedge for garnish

Instructions: Peel and grate the ginger. Cut the lemongrass into small pieces. Add the ginger and lemongrass to a glass with ice. Top with sparkling water. Squeeze the lime wedge into the glass and stir gently.

Preparation time: 5 minutes

Servings: 1

Mint and Elderflower Champagne Cocktail

Ingredients: 1 oz elderflower liqueur, 1/2 oz fresh lemon juice, 2 mint leaves, chilled champagne, mint sprig for garnish

Instructions: In a shaker, muddle the mint leaves. Add elderflower liqueur and lemon juice with ice. Shake until well combined. Strain into a champagne flute. Top with chilled champagne. Garnish with a mint sprig.

Preparation time: 5 minutes

Servings: 1

Lavender and Blueberry Mocktail

Ingredients: 1/2 cup blueberries, 1 oz lavender syrup, 1 oz fresh lemon juice, 4 oz sparkling water, lavender sprig for garnish

Instructions: In a glass, muddle the blueberries. Add ice, lavender syrup, and lemon juice. Stir gently. Top with sparkling water. Garnish with a lavender sprig.

Preparation time: 5 minutes

Servings: 1

Rosemary and Grapefruit Vodka Sour

Ingredients: 2 oz vodka, 1 oz rosemary simple syrup, 1 oz fresh grapefruit juice, 1 egg white, rosemary sprig and grapefruit wedge for garnish

Instructions: In a shaker, combine vodka, rosemary syrup, grapefruit juice, and egg white with ice. Shake vigorously for 15 seconds. Strain into a glass filled with ice. Garnish with a rosemary sprig and grapefruit wedge.

Preparation time: 10 minutes

Servings: 1

Herbal Beauty and Skincare Recipes

Lavender and Honey Face Mask

Ingredients: 1 tbsp dried lavender, 2 tbsp raw honey

Instructions: Grind the dried lavender into a powder using a mortar and pestle. Mix the lavender powder with raw honey. Apply the mixture to your face and leave it on for 10-15 minutes. Rinse with warm water.

Preparation time: 5 minutes

Servings: 1

Rose and Aloe Vera Face Toner

Ingredients: 1/2 cup rose water, 1/4 cup aloe vera gel, 1 tbsp witch hazel

Instructions: Mix all ingredients together and pour into a spray bottle. Shake well before each use. Spray onto your face after cleansing.

Preparation time: 5 minutes

Servings: 10

Peppermint and Tea Tree Oil Scalp Treatment
Ingredients: 2 tbsp coconut oil, 5 drops peppermint essential oil, 5 drops tea tree essential oil

Instructions: Melt the coconut oil and mix in the essential oils. Apply the mixture to your scalp and massage for 5-10 minutes. Leave it on for at least 30 minutes before washing your hair.

Preparation time: 10 minutes

Servings: 1

Chamomile and Lavender Eye Mask
Ingredients: 1/4 cup dried chamomile, 1/4 cup dried lavender, 1/2 cup rice

Instructions: Mix the dried chamomile and lavender with rice. Fill a small cloth bag with the mixture and tie the end. Heat in the microwave for 30 seconds and place over your eyes for 10-15 minutes.

Preparation time: 5 minutes

Servings: 1

Calendula and Shea Butter Body Balm
Ingredients: 1/4 cup dried calendula petals, 1/4 cup shea butter, 2 tbsp coconut oil, 5 drops lavender essential oil

Instructions: Infuse the dried calendula petals into the shea butter and coconut oil by placing them in a double boiler for 1-2 hours on low heat. Strain the mixture and let it cool until it solidifies. Mix in the lavender essential oil. Apply the balm to dry skin as needed.

Preparation time: 2 hours

Servings: 10

Turmeric and Honey Face Scrub

Ingredients: 1 tbsp ground turmeric, 2 tbsp raw honey, 1 tbsp coconut oil, 1 tbsp fine sea salt

Instructions: Mix all ingredients together to form a paste. Gently massage your face in circular motions for 2-3 minutes. Rinse with warm water.

Preparation time: 5 minutes

Servings: 1

Sage and Rosemary Hair Rinse

Ingredients: 1 cup apple cider vinegar, 1/4 cup fresh sage leaves, 1/4 cup fresh rosemary leaves

Instructions: Place the sage and rosemary in a jar and cover with apple cider vinegar. Let the mixture infuse for 1-2 weeks. Strain the herbs and pour the vinegar into a spray bottle. After shampooing, spray the vinegar onto your hair and scalp. Rinse with water.

Preparation time: 10 minutes

Servings: 10

Lavender and Chamomile Bath Soak

Ingredients: 1 cup Epsom salt, 1/4 cup dried lavender, 1/4 cup dried chamomile

Instructions: Mix all ingredients together and add to a warm bath. Soak for 20-30 minutes to relax and soothe your skin.

Preparation time: 5 minutes

Servings: 1

Green Tea and Lemon Facial Mist

Ingredients: 1 cup brewed green tea, 1/4 cup fresh lemon juice, 1/4 cup witch hazel

Instructions: Mix all ingredients together and pour into a spray bottle. Shake well before each use. Spray onto your face throughout the day for a refreshing boost.

Preparation time: 10 minutes

Servings: 10

Peppermint and Eucalyptus Foot Scrub

Ingredients: 1/2 cup coconut oil, 1/2 cup granulated sugar, 10 drops peppermint essential oil, 10 drops eucalyptus essential oil

Instructions: Mix all ingredients together to form a paste. Gently massage your feet in circular motions for 2-3 minutes. Rinse with warm water.

Preparation time: 5 minutes

Servings: 1

Calendula and Lavender Hand Salve

Ingredients: 1/4 cup dried calendula petals, 1/4 cup dried lavender, 1/2 cup coconut oil, 1/4 cup beeswax pellets

Instructions: Infuse the dried calendula petals and lavender into the coconut oil by placing them in a double boiler for 1-2 hours on low heat. Strain the mixture and return it to the double boiler. Add the beeswax pellets and heat until melted. Pour the mixture into a container and let it cool until it solidifies. Apply to dry hands as needed.

Preparation time: 2 hours

Servings: 10

Rose and Lavender Body Wash

Ingredients: 1/2 cup liquid castile soap, 1/4 cup dried rose petals, 1/4 cup dried lavender, 1 tbsp sweet almond oil, 5 drops rose essential oil, 5 drops lavender essential oil

Instructions: Infuse the dried rose petals and lavender into the sweet almond oil by placing them in a double boiler for 1-2 hours on low heat. Strain the mixture and mix with the liquid castile soap. Add the essential oils and stir to combine. Pour into a bottle and use as a body wash in the shower.

Preparation time: 2 hours

Servings: 10

Herbal Recipes for Health Conditions

Immune Boosting Tea

Ingredients:

1 teaspoon dried echinacea

1 teaspoon dried elderberry

1 teaspoon dried ginger

2 cups water

Instructions:

Add all the ingredients to a small saucepan and bring to a boil.

Reduce the heat and simmer for 10 minutes.

Strain the tea and serve hot.

Preparation time: 15 minutes

Servings: 2

Digestive Tea

Ingredients:

1 teaspoon dried peppermint

1 teaspoon dried chamomile

2 cups water

Instructions:

Add all the ingredients to a small saucepan and bring to a boil.

Reduce the heat and simmer for 10 minutes.

Strain the tea and serve hot.

Preparation time: 15 minutes

Servings: 2

Relaxation Tea

Ingredients:

1 teaspoon dried lavender

1 teaspoon dried lemon balm

2 cups water

Instructions:

Add all the ingredients to a small saucepan and bring to a boil.

Reduce the heat and simmer for 10 minutes.

Strain the tea and serve hot.

Preparation time: 15 minutes

Servings: 2

Headache Relief Tea

Ingredients:

1 teaspoon dried peppermint

1 teaspoon dried feverfew

2 cups water

Instructions:

Add all the ingredients to a small saucepan and bring to a boil.

Reduce the heat and simmer for 10 minutes.

Strain the tea and serve hot.

Preparation time: 15 minutes

Servings: 2

Cough and Cold Tea

Ingredients:

1 teaspoon dried thyme

1 teaspoon dried oregano

2 cups water

Instructions:

Add all the ingredients to a small saucepan and bring to a boil.

Reduce the heat and simmer for 10 minutes.

Strain the tea and serve hot.

Preparation time: 15 minutes

Servings: 2

Joint Pain Tea

Ingredients:

1 teaspoon dried turmeric

1 teaspoon dried ginger

2 cups water

Instructions:

Add all the ingredients to a small saucepan and bring to a boil.

Reduce the heat and simmer for 10 minutes.

Strain the tea and serve hot.

Preparation time: 15 minutes

Servings: 2

Nausea Relief Tea

Ingredients:

1 teaspoon dried peppermint

1 teaspoon dried chamomile

2 cups water

Instructions:

Add all the ingredients to a small saucepan and bring to a boil.

Reduce the heat and simmer for 10 minutes.

Strain the tea and serve hot.

Preparation time: 15 minutes

Servings: 2

Insomnia Tea

Ingredients:

1 teaspoon dried valerian root

1 teaspoon dried passionflower

2 cups water

Instructions:

Add all the ingredients to a small saucepan and bring to a boil.

Reduce the heat and simmer for 10 minutes.

Strain the tea and serve hot.

Preparation time: 15 minutes

Servings: 2

Anxiety Relief Tea

Ingredients:

1 teaspoon dried chamomile

1 teaspoon dried lemon balm

2 cups water

Instructions:

Add all the ingredients to a small saucepan and bring to a boil.

Reduce the heat and simmer for 10 minutes.

3. Strain the tea and serve hot.

Preparation time: 15 minutes

Servings: 2

Blood Sugar Balancing Tea

Ingredients:

1 teaspoon dried cinnamon

1 teaspoon dried fenugreek

2 cups water

Instructions:

Add all the ingredients to a small saucepan and bring to a boil.

Reduce the heat and simmer for 10 minutes.

Strain the tea and serve hot.

Preparation time: 15 minutes

Servings: 2

Allergy Relief Tea

Ingredients:

1 teaspoon dried nettle leaf

1 teaspoon dried peppermint

2 cups water

Instructions:

Add all the ingredients to a small saucepan and bring to a boil.

Reduce the heat and simmer for 10 minutes.

Strain the tea and serve hot.

Preparation time: 15 minutes

Servings: 2

Menstrual Cramp Relief Tea

Ingredients:

1 teaspoon dried raspberry leaf

1 teaspoon dried ginger

2 cups water

Instructions:

Add all the ingredients to a small saucepan and bring to a boil.

Reduce the heat and simmer for 10 minutes.

Strain the tea and serve hot.

Preparation time: 15 minutes

Servings: 2

Herbal Recipes for Kids

Chamomile and Honey Tea

Ingredients:

1 tablespoon dried chamomile flowers

1 teaspoon honey

1 cup water

Instructions:

Bring water to a boil in a small pot.

Add chamomile flowers and reduce heat to low. Let simmer for 5 minutes.

Remove from heat and strain into a mug.

Stir in honey and serve.

Preparation time: 10 minutes

Servings: 1

Lavender Lemonade
Ingredients:

1/4 cup dried lavender flowers

1 cup fresh lemon juice

3/4 cup honey

5 cups water

Instructions:

In a large pot, bring 3 cups of water to a boil.

Add lavender flowers and honey, stirring until honey is dissolved.

Remove from heat and let steep for 30 minutes.

Strain the mixture into a pitcher.

Add lemon juice and remaining 2 cups of water.

Stir and refrigerate until chilled.

Preparation time: 45 minutes (including steeping time)

Servings: 6-8

Herbal Iced Tea
Ingredients:

1 tablespoon loose herbal tea (such as peppermint, lemon balm, or hibiscus)

4 cups water

1-2 tablespoons honey (optional)

Ice cubes

Instructions:

Bring water to a boil in a large pot.

Remove from heat and add herbal tea.

Let steep for 5-10 minutes.

Strain the mixture into a pitcher.

Stir in honey, if desired.

Refrigerate until chilled.

Serve over ice.

Preparation time: 15 minutes (including steeping time)

Servings: 4

Rosemary Roasted Potatoes
Ingredients:

2 pounds of baby potatoes

2 tablespoons fresh rosemary, chopped

1 tablespoon olive oil

Salt and pepper, to taste

Instructions:

Preheat oven to 400°F.

Cut potatoes in half and place in a large mixing bowl.

Add chopped rosemary, olive oil, salt, and pepper.

Toss to coat potatoes evenly.

Transfer potatoes to a baking sheet.

Roast for 30-40 minutes or until potatoes are tender and golden brown.

Serve hot.

Preparation time: 45 minutes

Servings: 4-6

Dandelion Salad
Ingredients:

4 cups dandelion greens, washed and chopped

1/4 cup walnuts, chopped

1/4 cup dried cranberries

2 tablespoons olive oil

1 tablespoon apple cider vinegar

Salt and pepper, to taste

Instructions:

In a large mixing bowl, combine dandelion greens, walnuts, and dried cranberries.

In a separate small bowl, whisk together olive oil, apple cider vinegar, salt, and pepper.

Pour dressing over salad and toss to coat evenly.

Serve immediately.

Preparation time: 10 minutes

Servings: 2-4

Cinnamon Apple Chips
Ingredients:

2-3 apples, thinly sliced

1 tablespoon ground cinnamon

1 tablespoon coconut oil

1 tablespoon honey (optional)

Instructions:

Preheat oven to 200°F.

In a small bowl, mix together cinnamon, coconut oil, and honey (if using).

Brush mixture onto both sides of apple slices.

Place apple slices in a single layer on a baking sheet.

Bake for 2-3 hours or until the chips are crispy and golden brown.

6. Let cool before serving.

Preparation time: 10 minutes (plus baking time)

Servings: 4-6

Lemon and Thyme Chicken
Ingredients:

4 boneless, skinless chicken breasts

1/4 cup olive oil

1/4 cup fresh lemon juice

2 tablespoons fresh thyme leaves

Salt and pepper, to taste

Instructions:

Preheat oven to 375°F.

In a small bowl, whisk together olive oil, lemon juice, thyme, salt, and pepper.

Place chicken breasts in a baking dish.

Pour marinade over the chicken, making sure each piece is coated.

Bake for 25-30 minutes or until chicken is cooked through.

Let cool for a few minutes before serving.

Preparation time: 35 minutes

Servings: 4

Ginger and Honey Glazed Carrots
Ingredients:

1-pound carrots peeled and sliced

2 tablespoons fresh ginger, grated

2 tablespoons honey

1 tablespoon butter

Salt and pepper, to taste

Instructions:

In a large pot, bring salted water to a boil.

Add sliced carrots and cook for 5-7 minutes or until tender.

Drain and set aside.

In a small saucepan, melt butter over medium heat.

Add grated ginger and cook for 1-2 minutes.

Stir in honey and continue to cook for another 1-2 minutes.

Pour glaze over cooked carrots and toss to coat evenly.

Serve hot.

Preparation time: 20 minutes

Servings: 4-6

Mint Chocolate Chip Smoothie
Ingredients:

2 cups almond milk

1 banana, peeled and frozen

1/4 cup fresh mint leaves

1/4 cup dark chocolate chips

1 tablespoon honey (optional)

Instructions:

In a blender, combine almond milk, frozen banana, fresh mint leaves, and chocolate chips.

Blend until smooth.

Taste and add honey if desired.

Pour into glasses and serve immediately.

Preparation time: 10 minutes

Servings: 2

Turmeric Golden Milk
Ingredients:

2 cups unsweetened almond milk

1 teaspoon ground turmeric

1/2 teaspoon ground cinnamon

1/4 teaspoon ground ginger

1 tablespoon honey (optional)

Pinch of black pepper

Instructions:

In a small saucepan, heat almond milk over medium heat.

Add turmeric, cinnamon, ginger, honey, and black pepper.

Whisk to combine.

Cook for 3-5 minutes or until heated through.

Pour into mugs and serve hot.

Preparation time: 10 minutes

Servings: 2

Blueberry Oatmeal Bars
Ingredients:

1 cup rolled oats

1/2 cup almond flour

1/4 cup coconut oil

1/4 cup honey

1 teaspoon vanilla extract

1/4 teaspoon salt

1 cup fresh blueberries

Instructions:

Preheat oven to 350°F.

In a large mixing bowl, combine oats, almond flour, coconut oil, honey, vanilla extract, and salt.

Mix until a dough forms.

Fold in fresh blueberries.

Press the mixture into a greased 8x8 baking dish.

Bake for 20-25 minutes or until golden brown.

Let cool before slicing into bars.

Preparation time: 10 minutes (plus baking time)

Servings: 8-10

Rosemary Roasted Potatoes
Ingredients:

2 pounds of baby potatoes, halved

2 tablespoons olive oil

1 tablespoon fresh rosemary leaves, chopped

Salt and pepper, to taste

Instructions:

Preheat oven to 400°F.

In a large mixing bowl, toss potatoes with olive oil, rosemary, salt, and pepper.

Transfer potatoes to a baking sheet and spread them out in a single layer.

Bake for 25-30 minutes or until potatoes are crispy and golden brown.

Let cool for a few minutes before serving.

Preparation time: 10 minutes (plus baking time)

Servings: 4-6

PART 03

Chapter 07　　Growing Medicinal Plants

Grown at home, medicinal plants are an easy way to supply yourself with the medicine you need without having to go out into the wild and hoping for a good harvest. You can easily grow herbs indoors by following these steps!

Why grow medicinal plants?

- To save money. Growing your own herbs and spices can be a great way to save money on expensive, store-bought products. And if you're feeling adventurous, try making your own herbal remedies!
- To learn more about the world around you. The more knowledge we have about our environment, the better prepared we are for its challenges and changes--and growing medicinal plants is one way of gaining this knowledge firsthand.

Benefits of growing medicinal plants

Growing medicinal plants is a great way to get started with gardening and natural medicine. It can be a very rewarding hobby, especially if you're interested in learning more about herbs and herbal remedies.

Here are some reasons why growing medicinal plants is beneficial: You can grow your own supply of herbs for use in cooking or making teas. Many types of medicinal plants are known for their beauty as well as their healing properties. It's easy to grow most herbs indoors during winter months when there isn't much sunlight available outside (or anywhere else).

The importance of sustainable cultivation practices

Sustainable cultivation is a growing trend in the medicinal plant industry. It's also a necessity for many reasons, including:

- Increased crop yields and quality
- Better soil and water quality
- Reduced use of pesticides and fertilizers

Choosing the Right Medicinal Plants to Grow

Choosing the right medicinal plants to grow is an important first step in your journey as a home gardener. Different plants have different growing requirements, so it's important that you choose the ones that are best suited for your particular climate and environment.

It's also important to consider how much time and effort you want to put into caring for your plants--some require more attention than others, depending on how much water they need or how often they need pruning or harvesting.

Understanding the different types of medicinal plants

Medicinal plants are the foundation of traditional medicine. They're used to treat a wide range of ailments, from headaches and colds to cancer and HIV/AIDS.

Medicinal plants fall into three categories: herbal supplements (which are made from dried or fresh plant materials), phytochemicals (chemicals found in plants that have medicinal properties), and whole herbs (whole dried or fresh plants used as medicine).

Factors to consider when choosing medicinal plants to grow

When you're choosing plants to grow, there are several factors you should consider.

- The quality of the soil in your area. If it's poor, or if it has been depleted from overuse and/or intensive farming methods, then it is likely that any plant grown in this soil will be less healthy than its counterparts grown in better-quality soil.
- Weather conditions during the growing season: whether too hot or too cold at certain times of year may affect how well a plant grows. For example, basil likes warmer temperatures than many other herbs, so if you live somewhere with cooler summers than most other places (like Colorado), basil might be more difficult for you to grow successfully compared with someone living somewhere like Florida, where basil grows naturally.

Popular medicinal plants to grow and their uses

There are many different types of medicinal plants and herbs that you can grow at home. They have a variety of uses, from treating common ailments to helping with digestion and even boosting your immune system. Here are some popular ones:

- Garlic - This pungent bulb contains allicin, which has been shown to improve cardiovascular health by reducing bad cholesterol levels and increasing good cholesterol levels in the blood. It also helps prevent blood clots by thinning the blood.
- Ginger - The root contains shogaols (gingerols) that help reduce nausea during pregnancy or motion sickness.

- Rosemary - This herb is used as an antioxidant when added to foods such as chicken or grilled vegetables (it's commonly added when cooking meat). Rosemary can also be used topically on wounds as it has antibacterial properties.

Preparing the soil for medicinal plant cultivation

The first step in growing medicinal plants is to prepare the soil. To do this, you will need:

- A shovel or trowel. The size of your tool depends on how much work needs to be done; a small garden can get by with a hand shovel, while larger gardens will require crowbars and pickaxes!
- A rake. This tool helps loosen up the soil so that it's easier for you and your plant's roots to penetrate it when they grow later on!

Planting techniques for medicinal plants

To ensure that your plants get off to a good start and grow strong, follow these tips:

- If you're starting from seeds, sow them in well-drained soil that has been enriched with compost or aged manure. The best way to do this is in trays of seed compost; make sure each seed has about 1/2" (1 cm) depth of soil above it. Water the tray until all the compost is moist but not soggy; then cover it with clear plastic wrap and place it in a warm spot out of direct sunlight until germination occurs (usually 2-3 weeks). Once they have germinated, remove any dead or weak-looking plants before transplanting them into larger pots filled with fresh potting mix so they can continue growing vigorously at this stage too!
- To help prevent disease while still maintaining healthy crops, try planting some basil around other crops such as tomatoes or strawberries--these herbs have natural chemicals called essential oils, which protect against fungal diseases like powdery mildew by making air passages harder for spores to reach their host plants.

Optimal growing conditions for medicinal plants

- Temperature: Medicinal plants grow best between 65- and 85 degrees Fahrenheit.
- Humidity: Plants need to be kept in humid environments that are between 40 and 60 percent relative humidity.
- Light: Most medicinal plants thrive with bright light, but they can also grow in partial shade or darkness if necessary.

Common pests and diseases and how to manage them

Pests and diseases can be a major problem for your medicinal garden. Here's what to do if you find yourself dealing with these common issues:

- Pest management: If you notice any pests in your herb garden, remove the plant from the soil and place it in a bucket of soapy water for 24 hours. Afterward, remove all affected leaves before replanting them back into their original spot.

- Disease management: To prevent diseases from spreading, always use a sterile potting mix when repotting plants or transplanting them into larger containers (to prevent root rot). You should also avoid overwatering because this leads to damping off disease, which attacks young seedlings at their base, causing them to collapse over time; instead, allow soil surface to dry between watering sessions by keeping container lids off during warm weather months when possible.

Pruning and training techniques for medicinal plants

Pruning and training techniques are used to control the size, shape, and habit of a plant. They can be used to encourage an upright habit in plants that tend to grow sprawled on the ground, such as mints and lavender. Pruning techniques include:

- Pinching - Pinching out growing tips at regular intervals will encourage branching from side shoots (axillary buds). This is done by pinching off new shoots before they reach 10cm (4in) high; this also prevents them from flowering too soon. The remaining tips will develop into branches with many leaves that produce more essential oil than those that have been pinched back.

Fertilizing and watering requirements for medicinal plants

- Watering

Water your plants regularly, but don't overdo it. Too much water can cause root rot and other fungal problems that will kill your plant. Check the soil every day to see if it needs watering by poking a finger in and feeling for moisture. If you're growing indoors or in an artificial environment like a greenhouse, you may need to water more often than you would if you were growing outdoors because there will be less air circulation inside those structures which means that less evaporation occurs.

- Fertilizing

As with watering requirements, too much fertilizer is just as bad as not enough! Excess fertilizer can kill off beneficial microorganisms in the soil that help break down organic matter into nutrients plants can absorb through their roots (and which also make up part of their microbiome). Aim for about 1/4 cup per gallon every two weeks; this should provide plenty of nutrients without going overboard on unnecessary additives like pesticides or herbicides!

Identifying and harvesting medicinal plants

- When you're ready to harvest your medicinal plants, be sure to do so in a way that preserves their value. For example, if you are growing an herb like mint or basil for its oil content, use a sharp knife or scissors and cut them just above ground level. Cutting too low will damage the root system and make it more difficult for your plant to grow back next year.

- If you are harvesting roots or tubers (such as carrots), dig them up carefully with a shovel so as not to damage them further than necessary by pulling on them when removing them from the soil.

Best practices for drying and storing medicinal plants

Drying medicinal plants is a simple process that can be done in your own home. It's important to remember that not all medicinal plants will dry well, and some may need to be dried in a different way than others.

- Place the herbs on trays or screens in an area with good air circulation and low humidity (50% or less). Make sure they aren't touching each other or anything else that might cause them to stick together when they dry out.

- If your herb has been cut into smaller pieces, place them on wax paper so they don't stick together while drying out; this also makes it easier for you when it comes time for storage!

- Keep your herbs under these conditions until they are completely dry--this could take anywhere from three days up to a week, depending on what type of plant material you're using.

Methods for making medicinal plant products

There are several methods for making medicinal plant products. The best way to start is by learning how to make tinctures. Tinctures are a liquid extract of the medicinal plant's essential oils, which are then taken orally or applied topically. The process involves soaking dried or fresh herbs in high-proof alcohol (anywhere from 75-100%) for a period of time, straining them out, and diluting them with water, if necessary, before storing them in dark bottles away from heat and light.

In addition to tinctures, there are also teas--either hot or cold--and salves made from ingredients like beeswax, coconut oil, and other fats/oils, as well as infused oils (i.e., olive oil).

Understanding the safety and effectiveness of homemade remedies

There are two main concerns when it comes to making your own herbal remedies. The first is safety, and the second is effectiveness. We'll address each of these concerns in turn.

Incorporating medicinal plants into your daily life

You can incorporate medicinal plants into your daily life in a number of ways. The most obvious is by taking herbal supplements, which are available at many health food stores and online. You can also make your own tinctures and teas using dried or fresh herbs; these methods are best suited for people with experience working with herbs, but they're easy enough to learn if you're willing to put in the time.

If you have an interest in learning more about how these plants affect our bodies, consider enrolling in a class on herbal medicine or botany (if available). Alternatively, there are plenty of books written about specific herbs that may be helpful as well!

Encouragement to get started with growing medicinal plants

If you are interested in learning how to grow medicinal plants, then this is the chapter for you! Growing your own medicinal plants can be a great way to ensure that you have access to them when needed. You may also want to consider growing some plants just for fun because they look nice or smell good.

In order for it all to work out properly, there are a few things that must be considered before starting your garden:

Herbs

Herbs are plants grown for their medicinal properties. They can be used to treat a variety of ailments, including coughs, colds, and stomach problems.

Herbs can be grown in your backyard or on a windowsill at home. Some herbs require more sunlight than others; check out our list below to find out which herbs thrive under different conditions!

Vegetables

Vegetable gardens are a great way to grow your own food without having to worry about pests or diseases, and they can be placed almost anywhere. Vegetables can be grown in containers on patios or balconies, as well as in larger gardens outside the home. Some vegetables are actually perennial plants that will come back year after year if you keep them happy--this means you won't have to start from scratch each spring!

Fruit Trees and Berries

Fruit trees and berries are a great way to get your hands on some tasty, healthy food. Fruit trees can also be used as ornamentals, so if you have limited space in your garden or yard and want to grow something edible, fruit trees might be a good choice!

Fruit tree varieties include apple; apricot; cherry; peach; pear; plum (European); quince (European). Berries include boysenberry; elderberry (red); gooseberry (European); raspberry

Grains and Seeds

- Grains and seeds. These are a good option if you want to grow your own food but don't have enough space for a full garden. They're also great if you want to save money by buying in bulk and growing your own food instead of buying it at the grocery store.
- Herbs and spices. If you're interested in making your own herbal remedies or making sure that the herbs used in cooking taste as fresh as possible, then growing these plants is a great idea!

Growing medicinal plants at home

Growing medicinal plants at home is a great way to save money and learn about herbs. You may be surprised by how easy it is to grow your own medicinal plants.

There are many different types of medicinal plants that can be grown in your garden or backyard, including:

- Alfalfa (Medicago sativa) - A plant used for its nutritional value as well as its ability to help cleanse the body of toxins. It's also used as an herbal supplement for digestive issues like irritable bowel syndrome (IBS). This herb is typically eaten raw but can also be cooked lightly with oil and seasoning.
- Calendula (Calendula officinalis) - Also known as pot marigold or common marigold, this annual flower has been used throughout history for treating many ailments, including acne, burns, and wounds, because of its anti-inflammatory properties

How to get started

- First, you'll need to make sure that you have a garden. This can be as simple as a few pots on your patio or as elaborate as an entire plot of land where you grow all kinds of plants. Either way, it should be somewhere that gets sunlight and has space for your medicinal plants to grow in their natural environment without being disturbed by other things like pests or disease-carrying insects.
- Next, if you want them to thrive, they will need plenty of water, so make sure there's always enough rainfall from either natural sources (rain) or manmade ones (sprinklers).

Grow herbs from seed.

You can grow herbs from seed, but you'll need to start the seeds indoors and transplant them outside when they're about 6 weeks old. You'll also want to keep your plants well-watered and mulched.

How to grow medicinal plants from cuttings

Cuttings are the easiest way to propagate plants. You can take cuttings from any plant, but it's best to use a healthy young one. The best time to do this is in spring or fall when the sap is flowing and less likely to be damaged by cold temperatures.

The best way to make a cutting is by using sharp scissors or pruners and making clean cuts just below a node (the place where leaves attach). Place your cuttings into pots filled with soil mix made for growing herbs and cover them with plastic wrap until they sprout new roots on their own, which should take about two weeks if conditions are right!

When to start gardening

The best time to start your medicinal plant garden is when you have the time and energy to maintain it. If you're busy with work or school, then spring may not be the best season for starting a new project like this. However, if there's no other time in which you can dedicate yourself fully towards caring for your plants (and maybe even harvesting some fresh herbs!), then go ahead and give it a shot!

Growing plants indoors is an easy and efficient way to supply yourself with the medicine you need without having to go out into the wild and hoping for a good harvest.

Growing your own medicinal plants isn't just for experts; it's also an excellent way for beginners to get started with growing their own medicine.

The first step in successfully growing medicinal plants is choosing the right place for them. The best location is one that's sunny and exposed to plenty of wind but not too hot or cold. A south-facing wall or fence can be ideal as long as it gets enough sunlight throughout the day and isn't blocked by trees or other buildings. If you have no choice but to grow your medicinal herbs indoors, make sure they get at least six hours per day of direct sunlight through a window.

Once you've chosen your space, you should begin preparing it by removing any junk from it and cleaning it thoroughly. Once you have done this, the next step is to prepare the soil for planting. To do this, dig up an area about one foot deep and then fill it with compost or manure. If there's no room in your backyard for a garden bed, then consider building one out of wood pallets.

- The next step is to create a potting mixture that is rich in nutrients and free of any harmful chemicals.
- To make your own, you'll need to combine equal amounts of topsoil or potting soil with peat moss or composted manure; add some bone meal and blood meal for added nutrients, then mix it all together in an open container with enough water to wet the mixture thoroughly but not so much that it's soggy.

Place your plants into the soil so that their roots are evenly spread out. You should be able to see a few inches of root on each side of the stem and no more than a few inches of stem above ground.

If you want to give them an extra boost, add some organic fertilizer or compost to help them get established in their new home.

At this point, you're probably thinking that growing medicinal plants is a lot harder than it sounds. And you're right! But don't worry--it's not impossible. Your plants will need the right conditions in order to grow properly and produce the medicine that you want them to make.

You can easily grow herbs indoors by following these steps!

Follow these steps to grow herbs in your home:

- Choose a sunny spot for your herbs. If you don't have one, try placing them near a window that gets lots of sunlight.
- Plant the seeds or seedlings in soil that drains well and is rich in organic material such as compost or manure. Make sure to water them regularly so they don't dry out!

If you're looking for a way to get more herbs in your life and increase your health and wellness, then growing them is the perfect solution. The best part about it is that it doesn't require any special skills or expertise--all you need is some soil and water! If you want to start growing medicinal plants at home, our guide will walk through all of the steps required for success.

PART 04

Chapter 08 Collecting medicinal plants

Once you've found a plant, it's time to collect it. To do this, you need to use your knife or scissors and cut off branches or leaves from the plant. Then put them into a plastic bag (or other container) so they don't dry out before you can take them home and add them to your collection.

Collecting is easy! You must remember not to pull too hard on the plant because that might damage its roots; instead, gently tug at it until it detaches from its stem or branch. The best place for collecting is in wild areas where there are lots of plants growing together--this way, there will be plenty of choices without having to walk very far from home!

Harvesting

Harvesting plants is an essential step in the process. It's best to do this during the plant's flowering stage, which will be indicated by flowers and/or fruit. The plant will also be at its strongest at this time, so it will yield more useful ingredients than if you harvest earlier or later in its life cycle.

Once you've chosen which plants to collect, make sure they meet these criteria:

- They're not poisonous or toxic (you can tell by looking at their leaves)
- They don't have any large bugs on them

Medicinal plants are some of the most important for human health and well-being. They provide us with many valuable medicines we wouldn't otherwise have access to. Many species are used for medicinal purposes, from trees and flowers to herbs and spices—and they all play an essential role in the medical industry. It's estimated that 90 percent of drugs sold today were derived from plants first used by traditional healers thousands of years ago! These natural remedies offer several advantages over conventional medicines: they're often easier on your body because they're made with fewer chemicals; they can be grown on marginal land with less water and less fertilizer than cotton or sugarcane; and they can be produced at a lower cost than conventional crops like wheat or corn (which requires fertilizers). However, this doesn't mean that using medicinal plants is without problems—many species are threatened by extinction due to climate change (including deforestation), overharvesting by wild collectors/farmers who don't know what their impact might be on their environment (such as harvesting too much plant material), lack of demand in emerging economies where pharmaceutical companies cannot afford the high costs associated with research plus production costs necessary for launching drugs onto market shelves (bottom line profits matter more than helping people stay healthy)."

They can be used as medicines, food, cosmetics, and building materials. Medicinal plants provide a wide range of benefits for people worldwide, including alternative treatments for diseases that are difficult or impossible to treat using conventional methods.

Medicinal plant conservation is the protection of the genetic resources of medicinal plants through sustainable use by local communities or by commercial interests to ensure availability in the future for present and future generations.

Many of the world's medicinal plants are threatened by extinction.

These include:

- Artemisia annua (sweet wormwood) has been used as a treatment for malaria since ancient times. It is now cultivated in China, but wild populations have declined due to over-harvesting and habitat loss.
- Rauwolfia serpentina (snakeroot) is another important source of medicines used in Ayurvedic medicine in India, where it is effective against hypertension and epilepsy. However, its numbers have declined due to deforestation in its native Bhutan and India.

Conservation efforts can help protect medicinal plants.

- There are many ways of conserving and protecting medicinal plants, including:

• Saving seeds and replanting them in new areas. This is called seed banking.

• Growing the plant in controlled conditions so that you don't have to worry about it being destroyed by weather or pests. This is called cultivation or cultivation banking.

The conservation of medicinal plants is critical to human health.

Plants are our first and most powerful allies in the fight against disease, with the potential to heal us from within by boosting our immune system or providing relief from symptoms like inflammation. But these ancient cures will disappear forever if we don't care for them.

There are thousands of plant species used for medicinal purposes around the world, yet only about half have been studied by scientists for their effectiveness in treating diseases such as cancer and diabetes--and even fewer have been approved by regulatory agencies like the Food & Drug Administration (FDA). Some studies suggest that many herbal remedies may not be effective!

There is a growing demand for medicinal plants in the market.

The increasing population and the rising interest in traditional medicine have increased the demand for medicinal plants. This has made many companies move towards organic farming methods, which not only help preserve these plants but also ensure that they are grown without any chemicals or pesticides used on them.

The government needs to develop policies to help conserve these species and ensure they are sustainably harvested to ensure their availability even after we're gone!

The use of medicinal plants is an age-old practice.

It's no secret that the world has become increasingly dependent on synthetic drugs and medications. However, there is still a place for natural remedies in modern medicine, which is growing daily.

Medicinal plants have been used for thousands of years to treat various ailments and conditions. In recent decades, there has been an increased interest in these plants due to their ability to help people treat diseases without side effects or harsh chemicals.

The use of medicinal plants offers several advantages over conventional medicines.

Medicinal plants offer several advantages over conventional medicines. First, they are typically cheaper and more readily available than synthetic drugs. Second, they are often safer than synthetic drugs because their chemical structures have been studied for centuries by generations of herbalists. Finally, many medicinal plants can be cultivated in the wild or on farmland without damaging the environment or displacing other species.

Medicinal plants are important for many industries. For example, the production of medicinal plants is not only important for medical science but also for other industries like food, textile, and cosmetics.

Growing medicinal plants on marginal land can be a viable alternative to conventional crops such as cotton and sugarcane.

Medicinal plants can be grown on marginal land with less water and fertilizer than conventional crops like cotton and sugarcane.

Many types of traditional medicine are made using various kinds of trees, flowers, and herbs in the country.

The use of these natural resources has been a part of our culture for centuries, and it's hard to imagine an Indian home without them.

Efficient use of medicinal plants

The sustainable use of medicinal plants is important for their conservation. The following measures can achieve this:

- Improved cultivation practices include non-chemical weed control, soil management, and crop rotation.

Conservation of medicinal plants

- Conservation is the protection of natural resources for future generations. It also refers to managing these resources so that they are used sustainably.
- Conservation includes biodiversity and ecosystem conservation, defined as "the maintenance of ecosystem services" and "the maintenance of genetic diversity," respectively. The term "conservation" may also refer to harvesting wild plants or animals (harvesting) for food or medicine without destroying them; alternatively, it can mean reducing human-caused damage to an area, like pollution control in air quality management programs.

Sustainability and conservation of wild-collected species

As with any natural resource, ensuring our products are sustainably sourced and harvested is important. This is particularly true for medicinal plants often collected from remote and fragile ecosystems. Wild populations have often declined due to overexploitation by commercial collectors, who harvest large quantities of the same species year after year without regeneration or long-term management plans

.

Conservation strategies have been suggested to maintain the supplies of medicinal plants and ensure their availability to people in need. These include:

- Identification and protection of wild populations of threatened species through education and legislation;
- Establishment of botanical gardens;
- Establishment of seed banks;

These measures can help ensure that future generations will benefit from these important medicinal plants.

Conservation strategies include the protection of plant populations and their habitats, cultivation in botanical gardens or field-testing sites, ex-situ conservation of germplasm (e.g., cryopreservation), and the sustainable use of wild-collected plant material.

The most effective way to conserve plants is through protection of their habitats. In some cases, this can be achieved by establishing protected areas where plants grow naturally. Still, for many species that occur outside protected areas, such as rainforests, it may be necessary to create new land reserves specifically for them or restore degraded habitats so that it can once again support these rare species.

Governments and international agencies acting to protect these plants increasingly recognize the need for the conservation and sustainable use of medicinal plants.

However, many species used for medicinal purposes still need to be cultivated by farmers, who often live far from markets. They depend on harvesting wild-growing plants or gathering them from forests or other natural habitats. This can lead to unchecked overharvesting and habitat destruction; it also threatens the livelihoods of indigenous people who depend on these resources for survival.

There is concern that if all these factors work together against efforts to conserve medicinal plants, then we may lose some valuable medicines forever.

The main reason medicinal plants are becoming extinct is land use changes. The demand for food and fuel has led to clearing forests for farming or other uses such as logging or mining. This has resulted in the loss of many species' natural habitats and led to their extinction as well as making them harder to find when they are needed by humans today.

The medical industry has relied on medicinal plants for centuries and continues to do so today. Medicinal plants are the source of many drugs in modern medicine, including aspirin, morphine, and Taxol (a drug used to treat cancer).

The use of medicinal plants is not only sustainable and economically viable but also environmentally friendly.

- There are many reasons why we should use medicinal plants instead of synthetic drugs:
- They're cheaper and more effective than synthetic drugs.
- They can be grown locally, reducing transportation costs and pollution from shipping them over long distances by air or sea.
- The biodiversity of the plant kingdom is so vast that it's unlikely we'll ever exhaust all its possibilities for new medicines (and even if we did exhaust all possible combinations of compounds within a single species, there are thousands more out there).

In order to conserve these plants, they must be harvested ethically.

These plants must be harvested ethically. This means that the harvesting of medicinal plants should not damage their habitat, and it should also be done without harming other species or people who live there.

According to the National Center for Biotechnology Information, out of 42 plant species used traditionally, only 20 percent are threatened with extinction. This is less than 1% of the total number of plants today.

Traditional medicine is based on the use of plants to treat ailments.

Medicinal plants have been a part of human history since ancient times, but there is still much to be discovered about how they work and how they can be used more effectively as medicine.

In this chapter, we'll look at some examples of how researchers are working to conserve these valuable resources while making them available for future generations.

This practice has been around for centuries.

The use of medicinal plants has been around for centuries, and it's not going away anytime soon. Many people believe we should be using them more than we do today.

This practice has been around for centuries. Many people believe we should be using them more than we do today!

In many of the world's population, traditional medicine still plays an essential role in their health care. For instance, some studies show that approximately 70 percent of people worldwide use plants as part of their primary healthcare regimen.

Modern medicine has only sometimes been able to address all of our health concerns.

The field of medicine is constantly evolving, but it has not always been able to address all of our health concerns. For example, many people in the United States today suffer from various forms of arthritis and other chronic pain conditions that can be difficult to treat. As a result, they may turn to alternative therapies such as acupuncture or massage therapy in an effort to find relief from their symptoms. These approaches are often effective at managing pain levels while also improving the overall quality of life for patients who have difficulty walking due to severe joint inflammation or stiffness--but they aren't always covered by insurance companies because they aren't considered "evidence-based."

In addition to helping people cope with physical symptoms like these caused by arthritis (or even just everyday aches), some herbs used in traditional medicine have been shown through scientific studies conducted over time all over Earth's continents how useful they are when it comes down

.

Medicinal plants are threatened by climate change and deforestation.

In a study published in Nature Plants, researchers found that the growing season had lengthened by an average of 1.2 days per decade since 1980. The warming trend has been associated with changes in rainfall patterns, affecting plant growth and reproduction rates.

In addition to rising temperatures, we're also seeing more extreme weather events such as droughts and flooding due to climate change--and these can have devastating effects on medicinal plants if they occur during crucial parts of their lifecycle (like flowering or seed production).

These plants need our help!

It's important to note that these plants are not endangered but at risk of extinction. That means they're in danger of being wiped out entirely if we don't care for them.

It's also worth mentioning that many medicinal plants are threatened by overharvesting and habitat destruction-- but there are ways you can help protect them!

Medicinal plants are essential to human health and well-being. They have been used for centuries and are integral to traditional medicine today. The production of medicinal plants is important for medical science and other industries such as agriculture, cosmetics, and pharmaceuticals.

- Store plants in a cool, dark place.
- Keep them away from heat and direct sunlight as much as possible.
- If storing your medicinal plants in an airtight container, ensure there is enough room for circulation so that the moisture levels don't get too high and cause mold or fungus growth on the plant material inside the container.

Preparing the plants

Once you've harvested your plant, it's time to prepare it. You can use a knife or scissors to cut off the leaves of a plant and dry them out in a paper bag or on a screen. If you're using an herb with flowers or fruit, pick these off first so they don't get crushed in transit.

If you want to store your herbs for later use, try drying them out in an oven set at 200 degrees Fahrenheit for about 15 minutes (or until they feel crispy). Another option is putting them on parchment paper and leaving them out overnight so that their moisture evaporates from their surfaces.

Learn to identify plants.

The first step to collecting medicinal plants is learning how to identify them. If you're hoping to use plants for their healing properties, you must know what you're working with so that your treatments are effective and safe.

Learning how to identify plants can be difficult at first, but don't worry--it gets easier with practice! There are many resources available online that will help guide you through the process of learning about different types of plants and their uses.

One great place where I learned about herbs was my local library; they had books on just about every kind of plant imaginable! You could also try asking your friends or family members who may have experience with growing things in their backyard gardens--they might even let you borrow some seeds or cuttings so that when spring comes around again next year (or whenever else), there'll already be some new additions waiting in the ground by then!

When you find a new plant, record its location.

- Keep a journal of the plants you collect.
- Write down where you found each plant, including GPS coordinates. This will help you remember where to find them again in future seasons or years, and it will be useful if other people want to look for the same plant in that area.

Use only a small amount of your harvest.

You do not have to use all of your harvest.

It's important to remember that you can only collect a few plants at a time, so it's best only to use what you need and save the rest for another day.

Harvest around the edge of a group of plants rather than directly from the center.

When harvesting a plant, cut it in such a way that you leave some of the roots intact. This will allow the plant to regenerate and grow back quickly. If you harvest directly from the center of a group of plants, they may only have time to recover after winter comes around again.

Make sure you know what you are doing before you try it.

- You should always know what you are doing before trying it.
- Be careful not to get your hands or face near the plants since they may be poisonous.
- If you have health problems or allergies, try this only if your doctor says so first!

Be respectful and take care not to damage the plants or their surroundings.

It's important to be respectful of the plants and their surroundings. When harvesting, avoid damaging the roots and stems of the plant as much as possible. If you need to cut off part of a plant, ensure that you do so with clean cuts; this will help prevent infection or disease from spreading into your collection.

When collecting in an area where many medicinal plants are growing close together, try not to disturb them too much by walking through them or picking up large quantities at once--you may even want to wear gloves if possible! This will help ensure that these valuable resources continue to thrive well into the future so they can provide us with medicine now and into the future.

- Respectful plant collectors will avoid damaging their subjects or habitat and take only what they need for themselves or their communities.
- They may also leave some plants behind to allow others to thrive.

What to look for in plants

The first thing to know is that not all plants are safe to eat. The key ingredients in medicinal plants are usually found in their roots, stems, leaves, and flowers--and sometimes even the bark of trees. Some plants may be poisonous if consumed in large quantities or by certain people (for example, pregnant women).

So, when looking for a plant that might help with your symptoms, avoiding any leaves with discoloration or signs of mold growing on them is best. Also, watch out for flowers eaten off by insects and animals; these will contain less medicinal value than those left untouched by critters!

Using your medicinal plants

When you're ready to use your medicinal plants, ensure you have the right equipment. You'll need the following:

- A mortar, pestle, or other grinding device (if you don't already have one). If possible, use a pestle made from stone or wood rather than metal-- can react negatively with some plant materials.
- A bowl or cup to hold the ground material while it dries out completely in direct sunlight. The bowl should be large enough so that the plant matter doesn't overflow when being ground up but small enough that there's room for a top lid (you'll need this later).

If you have one available, you can also use an airtight jar; just make sure not to put any water inside! This will keep things dry so nothing gets moldy before they're ready for storage in jars or bottles later on down the line...

Collecting medicinal plants is a stimulating activity for both adults and children.

The thrill of finding a new plant or discovering something that you didn't know about before can make you feel like a little kid again!

It can be a learning experience that brings the whole family together.

- You may be surprised to learn that your children are just as interested in collecting medicinal plants as you are, and it can be a learning experience that brings the whole family together.
- If you think of your yard or garden as an outdoor classroom, there is no limit to the number of things they can discover while they play outdoors.
- Take advantage of their natural curiosity by having them help gather some herbs, roots, and leaves from around the yard.

Taking suitable safety precautions is important if you are new to collecting plants.

- Wear long sleeves and pants. Keep your arms and legs covered to protect yourself from poison ivy, stinging nettles, or other harmful plants.
- Bring a water bottle on your hike to stay hydrated while collecting plants in the wild (or even at home). It's also good practice to carry a snack with you when out in nature; this will help keep hunger pangs at bay so that they don't distract from what matters most--your collection!

You need to know what you are doing, or you could damage the plant and lose its healing properties!

There are many things to consider when collecting medicinal plants. You need to know what you are doing, or you could damage the plant and lose its healing properties!

If you have picked flowers from your garden for a bouquet or cut down branches for use in a wreath, you have collected plants. This can be done as part of an educational program with children or adults interested in learning more about their local environment.

When gathering medicinal plants, it is crucial that you don't collect too many plants from one spot. This can cause harm to the ecosystem in which they grow.

It is also important not to remove all of one plant species' flowers or leaves at once, as this could lead to its extinction and make it harder for future generations to use these plants for medicine.

If you're interested in exploring medicinal herbs and how to use them, there are many resources online to help get you started!

There are many ways to teach kids about medicinal herbs without collecting them yourself.

- Read books together, like The Healing Herbs Garden or The Plant Doctor's Guide to Garden Remedies. These books are great for all ages and can be found at your local library or bookstore.
- Create a seed kit with seeds from the plants you want to grow in your garden and send it to a friend who needs some cheering!
- If your child wants a plant but not necessarily the whole mess of roots, bulbs, stems, and leaves that go along with it (or if you don't have room for all those things), try cutting off just one leaf from each plant instead--they're easy enough to keep alive indoors until springtime comes around again next year.

People have used the herbs and plants around them for thousands of years. They knew certain plants would help with their illnesses or injuries, so they collected them and prepared them differently. Some people used these herbs to make medicine, while others used them to dye their clothes or food. Plants can be beneficial in many ways!

There are many ways to gather wild medicinal plants. The most common is to pick the flowers, leaves, or stems and dry them in a cool, dark place. You can also make a tincture by soaking your plant material in alcohol for several weeks before straining it out and using the liquid as needed.

Other ways of preserving medicinal plants include freezing or preserving them in glycerin so they don't go wrong when exposed to air over time.

There are also times when you shouldn't gather wild plants.

- Don't pick flowers or leaves that are in bloom, as they're most likely to be pollinated at this time and will produce seeds. This can interfere with the plant's ability to reproduce itself in the future if harvested too heavily.
- Don't harvest anything sprayed with pesticides or fertilizers (unless it says "organic"). These chemicals can be detrimental to your health, not just because they are harmful but also because they may cause allergic reactions if ingested by humans or animals who eat them later on down the line.

Gathering medicinal plants can be safe, but there are some things you need to know first.

- Wear long pants and closed-toed shoes when you're out in the field. You don't want to get bitten by a snake or stung by a bee!

- If you're going on an extended hike or expedition, pack extra water and snacks if your walk takes longer. You'll also want to bring some first aid supplies like bandages, antiseptic wipes (like hydrogen peroxide), gauze pads/strips for wound dressing, tweezers for removing splinters--the list goes on!
- Always wear sunblock with SPF 30 or higher if you're going out during the day; this will protect against harmful UV rays, which can cause skin cancer later in life if overexposed over time without protection from them now while young enough still where it matters most.

Wildcrafting is collecting herbs from the wild and using them for medicinal purposes.

Wildcrafting can be both an ancient art and a modern science, depending on your perspective.

In fact, many people believe that we've been using wildcrafted herbs since humans first learned how to pick up sticks and walk upright. Others argue that it wasn't until European settlers arrived in America that they started harvesting plants from forests and fields with any regularity--and even then, only selectively: The colonists were looking for particular medicinal properties within each plant species rather than trying their luck at random.

Either way, our ancestors understood the value of natural remedies long before we did!

They're a great alternative to pharmaceutical drugs, which can be expensive and have side effects.

The medicinal properties of some plants are well known, but others haven't been studied as much and might not have been used traditionally by your community. To find out if native medicines could help you, ask an elder or tribal member in your area if they know anything about them.

Some people consider herbal medicine more natural or ecologically sound than modern medicine because it is made from plants and animals that are found in nature rather than chemicals produced in laboratories.

This belief is supported by the fact that many herbs used in traditional Chinese medicine were discovered thousands of years ago and have been used ever since without any harmful side effects being reported.

Other people think it is better not to disturb nature and that plenty of herbal remedies can be purchased at health food stores.

You may want to consider both points of view before deciding which way you want to go.

Herbalism is an old form of medicine, but it may not work as well as modern medicine.

Herbalism is a form of medicine used for thousands of years. It's still used today but might not be as effective as modern medicine.

Some herbal medicines are effective in treating certain diseases and conditions. For example, studies have shown that ginseng can help people with high blood pressure and diabetes mellitus. However, when we look at other herbal remedies like garlic or echinacea, we don't see any evidence that they work for treating anything other than colds.

There are benefits and drawbacks to charging medicinal plants in the wild.

If you have been practicing your herbalism skills, you know many different types of medicinal plants can be used for healing. Some of these plants may grow in your backyard or outside your door! However, suppose you don't have no experience harvesting these herbs yourself. In that case, it might be best for beginners to stick with grocery store-bought options until they learn how best to prepare them for consumption (and what precautions should be taken).

In the end, collecting medicinal plants is an excellent activity for both adults and children. It can be a learning experience that brings the whole family together, and it's also fun! If you're new to collecting plants, taking the right safety precautions is essential. You need to know what you are doing, or you could damage the plant and lose its healing properties. It is also important that you don't collect too many plants from one spot, as this can cause harm to the ecosystem in which they grow.

Chapter 09   Processing medicinal plants

Medicinal plants have been used for centuries by people around the world for their healing benefits. Plant medicine is an exciting topic combining art and science to produce herbal remedies with optimal health benefits.

Medicinal plants are used for their therapeutic value.

Medicinal plants are used for their therapeutic value. They're used to treat a wide range of illnesses, including chronic diseases and conditions like diabetes, hypertension and depression.

Medicinal plants can be consumed in different forms: fresh; dried; powdered; as an extract (liquid or solid), or tincture (alcohol-based solution).

The process of converting medicinal plants into extracts or oils is called phytochemicals.

Phytochemicals are the chemical compounds in plants responsible for their color, taste, and smell. These phytochemicals also have a variety of health benefits. Phytochemicals can be extracted from medicinal plants using various methods, including water or alcohol extraction (called extracts).

In addition to extracting phytochemicals from medicinal plants, you can use heat or pressure to convert them into oils. This process is called decarboxylation, which gives cannabis its psychoactive properties when smoked or vaporized.

Phytochemicals from plants work by targeting specific parts of the body and system, which help treat various ailments.

For example, phytochemicals that target the liver may be used to treat hepatitis or cirrhosis. Phytochemicals that target the lungs may be used for asthma or other lung conditions such as COPD (chronic obstructive pulmonary disease).

Phytochemicals are natural compounds in plants that provide health benefits beyond vitamins and minerals. Phytochemicals are the "extra" nutrients that help your body stay healthy. They work with other nutrients, such as vitamins and minerals, to protect cells from damage and fight disease.

There are thousands of different phytochemicals--so many that scientists haven't even identified them all yet! Some examples include:

- Flavonoids (found in fruits)
- Polyphenols (found in coffee)

In addition to their direct effects on the body, phytochemicals promote good gut function. Some of them are even thought to help the body produce its antioxidants and vitamins. Because of this, you must choose supplements that contain only high-quality ingredients--and avoid those with filler ingredients like soy lecithin or stearic acid (which may be derived from animal fat).

While it's true that all plants contain phytochemicals, not all phytochemicals are created equally. Many of them are destroyed during processing and extraction, so only those that are appropriately extracted will give you optimal benefits.

There is no one-size-fits-all approach to herbal remedies, but most agree that mixing different herbs increases their effectiveness. For example, if you want an anti-inflammatory effect from your medicine cabinet, consider pairing ginger with turmeric or rosemary.

To avoid any potential adverse interactions between herbs and medications (or even food), always consult a doctor before taking new supplements or medicines while pregnant or breastfeeding.

The Dangers of Toxic Plants

The first thing to remember is that many toxic plants can make you sick or even kill you. Some of these are dangerous because they're poisonous, and others because they have harmful chemicals that irritate your skin or mouth.

Some examples include:

- Poison Ivy (Rhus radicans) - This plant contains an oil called urushiol which causes contact dermatitis in humans, resulting in painful blisters on your skin if you come into contact with it. It also has anti-inflammatory properties that may benefit arthritis sufferers if taken internally in small doses (1-2 grams). However, this amount would be challenging to measure accurately due to its large size (the leaves are about 12 inches long).

How to Identify a Safe Plant

Before picking plants, you need to know what's safe and what's not. Here are some things to look out for:

- Don't eat it if you're unsure of the plant's identity!
- Do not eat plants if sprayed with pesticides or other chemicals (such as fungicides).
- Avoid eating any plant that has white sap unless you know for sure that it does not have toxic compounds in its leaves or stems. White sap is usually a sign of alkaloids or other potentially harmful substances in those parts of the plant.

Determining the Best Time to Harvest a Plant

The best time to harvest a plant is when it has reached its peak of maturity and health. This is generally when the leaves are full and green, with no signs of wilting or yellowing. If you do not know what type of plant you are harvesting, it's best to consult an expert to identify which stage would be most beneficial for your needs.

It's also important not to harvest too early or too late; this can affect potency and quality.

How to Determine Whether or Not a Plant is Medicinal

Next, you need to determine if the plant is medicinal. This can be done by observing its physical characteristics and comparing it with other plants known for their healing properties. For example, if you notice that a certain plant has leaves similar to those of an herb like aloe vera or echinacea, then it's likely that this new find also has healing properties. You may also want to ask an experienced herbalist for help determining whether your newly discovered plant has medicinal value.

The Art of Processing Medicinal Plants

Processing medicinal plants is an art. It's a skill that must be honed over time, and many factors affect the quality of the final product. For example, if you choose to smoke your medicinal plants rather than eat them in their raw form (which we recommend), you'll want to ensure they are dry enough before putting them into your pipe or rolling papers. If not dried properly, some plants will produce an unpleasant taste and burning sensation on your tongue when smoked--and no one wants that!

The same goes for tinctures: if you don't allow enough time to steep correctly in alcohol or glycerin solutions before bottling them up for storage at room temperature (not refrigerated), their potency will suffer considerably well.

In short: processing medicinal plants requires attention to detail--but don't worry! We've got your back on this one!

There are many ways to process medicinal plants for optimal health benefits

The most common methods include:

- Decoctions, infusions, and tinctures
- Dry-heating (roasting) and wet-heating (steaming)

Traditional medicine

Traditional medicine is an ancient practice that uses herbs, plants, and other natural remedies to treat illness. It has been practiced for thousands of years by various cultures around the world. The use of medicinal plants dates back to prehistoric times when humans began collecting them from nearby forests or fields. Early civilizations used these plants as part of their healing rituals before they could understand how each one worked individually at a molecular level.

Ethnobotany

Ethnobotany is the study of plants humans use and their relationships with people. Ethnobiologists study the cultural uses, history, and evolution of these plants. Ethnobotanical research has been important in developing medicines for treating diseases such as malaria and diabetes mellitus type II (DMII), which affect millions worldwide annually.

Ethno-botanical studies can be conducted at any level: from individual plants to entire cultures; from medicinal plant species collected locally to those traded internationally; from single-species habitats to diverse ecosystems; from small groups of people living on remote islands with limited access to outside resources, all the way up through large population centers where modern medicine has made most traditional remedies obsolete due to overuse or misuse--or simply because they don't work anymore after years of being passed down orally through generations without being tested scientifically first!

Pharmacognosy

Pharmacognosy is the study of drugs and medicines derived from natural sources. It is a field that focuses on how plants and herbs can treat diseases, improve health, and enhance well-being.

Pharmacognosy includes identifying, isolating, characterizing, extracting, and purifying plant compounds with medicinal properties. These compounds are then used in medicines or other products such as dietary supplements or cosmetics.

Herbalism

Herbalism is the art and science of processing medicinal plants for optimal health benefits. Herbalists use herbs to treat, prevent, and cure illnesses by treating the root cause of disease rather than just symptoms.

Herbs can be used in various ways, including tinctures (liquid extracts), teas, syrups, and salves. They can also be applied topically or taken internally as an herbal supplement.

Herbal medicine is an ancient form of healing that can be traced back to Chinese, Egyptian, and Indian civilizations. Herbalists have used herbs for thousands of years to treat various illnesses and ailments.

Herbs are plants that are used as medicine or food additives. They come from all over the world, but most herbs grow in temperate climates such as North America, Europe, and Asia. Some common examples include sage, echinacea, and ginger root.

Herbs have been used for centuries by cultures around the world because they provide many health benefits without side effects like those caused by conventional medicines.

Medical researchers are exploring the use of plants for healing.

Medical researchers are exploring the use of plants for healing. Plants contain many active ingredients and nutrients that can promote health when taken in appropriate amounts. Some of these substances include:

- Phytochemicals, including polyphenols and antioxidants
- Vitamins and minerals
- Fiber

Why is it essential to process medicinal plants in the first place?

The answer is that many plants contain compounds that are difficult for our bodies to absorb and use. The processing of these plants helps increase their bioavailability, or how much of their nutritional value can be used by your body.

For example, some plants can be used to treat heart disease, and others can treat cancer. Some herbs can help you lose weight, while others can help you sleep better at night.

Here's a quick list of some common medicinal plant types:

- Herbs include things like rosemary or thyme; they're usually used in cooking but also have health benefits when taken in capsule form or tinctured with alcohol (or vinegar). Herbs are often thought to be less powerful than other forms of medicine because they don't contain active ingredients like flowers and roots, but this may not always be true! Some herbs have more concentrated levels than those found elsewhere on the tree or bush, where it grows naturally.

The benefits of medicinal plant processing

The benefit of this process is that it's an easy way to store medicinal plants and make them more digestible. The longer you leave your herbs to steep, the stronger they will become. When you're ready for a dose of medicine, strain the liquid through cheesecloth or muslin cloth into a separate container and use it as needed (be sure not to drink all of it at once). This can be stored in the fridge for up to two weeks without losing potency!

Processing and preparing medicinal plants properly can make all the difference.

Extracting active compounds from plant material requires care, attention to detail, and a little know-how. Just like cooking!

Processing medicinal herbs involves three main steps: drying, grinding/pulverizing, and decocting (extracting).

Many people want to use medicinal plants to improve their health, yet they don't know how to identify them or how to make them into medicine.

If you're one of these people, I have good news for you: this chapter will teach you everything that you need to know about processing medicinal plants for optimal health benefits.

If you are new to plant medicine, the best way to begin using it is by learning to find and process plants with the right characteristics for your needs. Once you've found a plant that seems like it might be helpful for your health or spiritual practice, it's time to start learning how to harvest from them.

You can find a wealth of information online about the uses of herbal medicines, but there's nothing like learning from people who have done what you're doing and succeeded at it!

When collecting medicinal plants, always be sure you are legally allowed to do so in your area. Some areas have bans on collecting certain plants, especially those which may be endangered or have overabundant populations.

If you're unsure about the legality of picking a particular plant in your area, check with local authorities before harvesting it. In addition to respecting the environment and other people's property rights, this will also help prevent legal problems from arising later on if something goes wrong (e.g., someone else sees what looks like "their" plant being taken away by someone else).

When considering which herbs to use for your herbal medicine practice, try incorporating plants from native habitats into your repertoire. This will fit nicely with wildcrafting, where practitioners get herbs from natural sources instead of buying them in stores or growing indoors.

It's also important to consider how a particular plant grows in its environment and what conditions are necessary for optimum growth. For example, some plants require precise sunlight exposure or soil type; others grow better when planted near other plants (called companion planting).

- You can learn how to use medical herbs by picking them yourself or finding an herb class that teaches practical medicine-making knowledge.

- There are many ways to learn about medicinal plants, including books and videos. Some people with experience with herbal medicine will offer classes in their homes or other locations.
- If you are interested in learning more about medicinal plants and their uses, many different resources are available online and offline (in print).

Plants as medicine

Plants are a rich source of phytochemicals, which are compounds that give plants their color, flavor, and medicinal properties. Phytochemicals can be found in all plant parts, including leaves, flowers, and seeds.

Phytochemicals have antioxidant properties that may help protect against chronic diseases such as heart disease and cancer; they also regulate immune function and inflammation response.

Processing plants for optimal benefits

Processing plants are preparing a plant or its parts to make them more easily digestible and/or bioavailable. The most common form of processing is drying, which removes moisture from the plant material, making it easier to store. In addition, other processing forms include decoction (boiling), maceration (soaking), fermentation, and extraction using solvents such as alcohol or water.

The benefits of medicinal plant therapy are many.

Medicinal plant therapy can help you:

- Feel more energized and less stressed
- Improve your digestion and overall health
- Reduce inflammation in the body (which is a major cause of disease)

For example, the active ingredients in a plant can be used to treat or prevent diseases such as cancer, diabetes, or substance abuse. These chemicals are often found in plants used for centuries by traditional healers. In some cases, scientists have identified the chemical composition of these plants but not their biological activity.

They can also be used to treat symptoms of the disease.

The healing power of herbs is well known, and they can also be used to treat disease symptoms. They have been used for thousands of years by people all over the world in traditional medicine. Herbs contain active ingredients that work with your body's natural defenses to help heal and prevent illness, so it's not surprising that they are often effective at treating common diseases like colds or coughs.

Some herbs may help you feel better when you're sick by reducing coughing fits and chest tightness and increasing mucus production so you can clear up congestion more easily. Some herbs also have anti-inflammatory properties that help reduce swelling in the nose or throat area (like eucalyptus), which may make breathing easier if those areas are inflamed due to allergies or sinusitis (sinus infection).

These health benefits come from the chemicals found in plants.

Medicinal plants are a vital part of the human diet. The chemical compounds found in medicinal plants have been shown to have a number of health benefits, including reducing inflammation, improving heart health and brain function, and even fighting cancer. These chemical compounds are phytochemicals or phytonutrients - plant nutrients that provide vitamins, minerals, and other nutritional value beyond what can be obtained from animal products alone.

These chemicals are known as phytochemicals or phytomedicines.

You may be wondering what a phytochemical is. A phytochemical is a natural chemical found in plants that has health benefits for humans. They're also called phytomedicines, which means "medicines from plants."

Phytochemicals have been used for thousands of years by traditional healers around the world as remedies for various ailments, including digestive disorders, infections, and even cancer. Scientists are now learning more about how these chemicals can be used as treatments for modern-day diseases such as heart disease or diabetes--and they're discovering that many of them work better than pharmaceutical drugs!

These phytomedicines can also be used topically in skin creams and hair conditioners.

You can also use medicinal plants topically, such as in skin creams and hair conditioners. The anti-inflammatory properties of arnica are well known, so it's not surprising that one study found that arnica extract helped reduce inflammation and pain associated with eczema.

You may be wondering, "What is so exciting about medicinal plants?" Well, they can both improve your health and also help your physical appearance!

For example, did you know that the antioxidant-rich fruit of the moringa tree has been shown to have anti-aging properties? This means that eating or drinking moringa leaves can help reverse the signs of aging in your skin by reducing fine lines and wrinkles.

Medicinal plants have been used in healing since humans first began.

People have relied on natural substances to treat illnesses and injuries for thousands of years. Many medicinal plants are still used as primary treatments for conditions such as cancer, heart disease, and diabetes.

Medicinal plants are also used to prevent illness by boosting the immune system or reducing inflammation ("antioxidant activity"). Some examples include:

Plants contain many chemical compounds that provide health benefits but can also be toxic.

Plants contain a wide range of chemical compounds that provide health benefits but also can be toxic. The key to getting the most out of your medicinal plant is knowing how to prepare it properly before consuming it.

A good place to start is learning about the different types of plants you can use for your remedies and how they are used traditionally in folk medicine. The next step is understanding what makes each plant unique so you know which ones will benefit you the most based on your symptoms or condition. Finally, once you've chosen which plants are right for your needs (and have identified their active compounds), learn how best to prepare them before consuming them--this will ensure that they're safe and effective as part of your treatment plan!

Some plants are safer than others to use as medicine.

The good news is that some plants are safer than others for medicine. For example, you should avoid using plants with:

- Toxic or poisonous components;
- High concentrations of alkaloids (a class of chemicals produced by plants). Alkaloids can be toxic and even fatal at high doses; and
- Consistently high levels of oxalates (a type of salt). Oxalates can cause kidney stones and other health issues if consumed in large amounts over time.

Not all medicinal plants are safe to eat or drink.

Some can be poisonous, and some can even kill you. If you use medicinal plants as medicine, you must know how to identify and use them correctly.

Processing can make some medicinal plants more effective and safer to consume.

Drying, crushing, and grinding herbs into powder form is called "decoction." This ancient method helps break down the tough cell walls found in many medicinal plants. It also increases their bioavailability--the number of active compounds absorbed by your body when you consume them.

Processing is important for the safety and efficacy of herbal remedies.

It's a good idea to process your herbs as soon after harvesting them as possible. This can be done by drying or freezing them for later use. Drying is a simple process that requires little more than air circulation and sunlight; however, if you live in an area where humidity levels are high year-round (such as Florida), it's best to freeze your plants instead--this will keep them fresher longer by slowing down decomposition.

PART 05

Chapter 10   Herbs for Health, Wellness, and Beauty

Herbs are nature's medicine. They're powerful, easy to use, and can help you feel better.

Overview of herbs and their benefits for health, wellness, and beauty

Herbs are plants that have been used for healing and nutritional properties for thousands of years. They can be found all over the world, growing wild or cultivated in gardens. Herbs have been used as medicine throughout history, and modern science has proved their effectiveness repeatedly. Herbs can be used in many different ways: as teas or tinctures (alcohol-based extractions), oils or lotions made from them, honey-based syrups called meads, etc. The uses of herbs vary depending on their properties; some herbs will help you relax, while others will invigorate you!

Importance of using herbs as a natural remedy

There are many benefits to using herbs as a natural remedy. Herbs can be used to treat a variety of conditions, including:

- Acne
- Allergies and asthma
- Anxiety disorders such as panic attacks or post-traumatic stress disorder (PTSD)
- Arthritis and joint pain
- Bronchitis, coughs, and colds
- Diabetes management

Herbs for digestive health (e.g., peppermint, ginger, chamomile)

Herbs beneficial for digestive health include peppermint, ginger, and chamomile.

Peppermint is known for its cooling and refreshing properties. It's a great herb when you're feeling bloated or sluggish after eating a large meal. You can drink peppermint tea with honey to soothe inflammation in the stomach as well as relieve indigestion. Peppermint also helps calm acid reflux by relaxing muscles in your esophagus that cause heartburn symptoms when they contract too frequently (source).

Ginger root has been used for centuries because of its anti-inflammatory properties; it relieves pain from acute inflammation (like an injury) and chronic inflammation (like arthritis). In addition to relieving pain associated with these conditions, ginger also stimulates circulation throughout the body, which increases blood flow around nerves--this helps improve mobility without causing any negative side effects like dizziness or nausea (source).

Herbs for pain relief (e.g., arnica, devil's claw, turmeric)

This section will cover some of the most popular herbs for pain relief. These include arnica, devil's claw, and turmeric.

- Arnica: This herb has been used for centuries to treat aches and pains associated with muscle injuries. It works by increasing blood flow to injured areas while decreasing inflammation simultaneously, which helps reduce swelling.
- Devil's Claw: The South African plant is traditionally used as an anti-inflammatory agent that can help reduce joint stiffness.
- Turmeric: This spice contains curcuminoids (a compound) that are thought to have anti-inflammatory benefits when taken orally.

Herbs for sleep (e.g., lavender, passionflower, hops)

Lavender

Lavender is a popular herb that can help you relax and sleep better. It's also known for its anti-inflammatory properties, which can help treat pain associated with arthritis or other conditions.

Passionflower

Passionflower has been a calming agent since ancient times and may help reduce anxiety, nervousness, and restlessness. This herb also improves sleep quality in people who have insomnia or other sleep disorders such as restless leg syndrome (RLS).

Hops

Hops are used in brewing beer but have long been valued for their medicinal properties as well; they've been used since medieval times as a folk remedy for insomnia because they contain compounds that act on the central nervous system in ways similar to prescription drugs like Valium but without many of their side effects.

Herbs for energy and focus (e.g., ginseng, Rhodora, maca)

In the quest for optimal health, wellness, and beauty, herbs can be a powerful ally. In this section, we'll explore some of the most popular herbs known to promote energy and focus.

- Ginseng: This root has been used in traditional Chinese medicine (TCM) for thousands of years as an herb that supports vitality and longevity. It's also an adaptogen because it helps your body deal with stress by balancing hormones like cortisol and boosting your immune system.

- Rho Diola: This flowering plant grows throughout Europe and Asia but is most abundant in cold climates such as Siberia or Scandinavia. Although it's sometimes called "golden root," Rhodora has red stems with yellow flowers--a pretty contrast against deep green leaves!

Herbs for skin care (e.g., aloe vera, calendula, chamomile)

Herbs are not only effective in maintaining general health and wellness but they can also be used to treat specific conditions such as acne or eczema. In addition to their medicinal properties, herbs have the added benefit of being gentle on the skin and often smell great!

Here are some examples of herbs that you may want to consider adding to your skincare routine:

- Aloe Vera - This plant has been used for thousands of years as a natural remedy for burns, wounds, and other skin problems. It contains vitamins A & C along with minerals such as zinc and potassium, which help repair damaged tissue while soothing inflammation at the same time. You can find this ingredient in many products, including lotions (which often contain additional ingredients like witch hazel), soaps/shampoos/conditioners, etc.

Herbs for hair care (e.g., rosemary, nettle, horsetail)

Have you ever wondered how to make your hair grow faster? If so, it's important to know that many herbs can help with this issue. Rosemary is an excellent example of an herb that can help with growing out your locks and making them healthier in general. This herb has been used for centuries by people around the world because of its powerful properties when it comes to caring for our bodies and minds. Rosemary contains antioxidants that help fight free radicals in our bodies, which may cause disease or cancerous cells to form on our skin or scalp area, where we apply this herb as a topical treatment.

Nettles have been used by many cultures around the world because they contain nutrients like vitamins A & C along with iron, among other minerals needed for optimal health, including zinc which helps boost energy levels while reducing fatigue when taken internally; iron builds up red blood cells so they carry more oxygen throughout our body helping us feel stronger overall physically while boosting mental clarity at the same time. Horsetail is another great option if you want healthy hair growth, too - especially if yours tends to break off easily due to stressors such as dieting too hard without enough protein intake per day (which happens all too often).

Herbs for overall beauty and anti-aging (e.g., green tea, gout kola, hibiscus)

- Green tea: green tea is high in antioxidants and polyphenols, which have been shown to have anti-inflammatory properties. These compounds have also been linked to lower rates of cancer, heart disease, and diabetes.

- Gout kola: Gout kola has been used for centuries to treat skin disorders such as acne and psoriasis. Research suggests it could help wound healing by promoting collagen production (a protein found in connective tissue). It's also said to improve circulation and reduce swelling around the eyes because it can regulate blood pressure levels while reducing stress hormones like cortisol or adrenaline/noradrenaline. Hibiscus: The flowers of this shrub are rich in tannins that act as astringents when applied topically-- meaning they tighten skin by constricting capillaries under the surface.

Precautions when using herbs (e.g., interactions with medications, allergies)

- Use herbs with caution if you're pregnant or breastfeeding.
- Some herbs can interact with medications or cause allergic reactions. If you are taking any prescription drugs, speak with your doctor before using herbal supplements to ensure they don't interfere with the effectiveness of the medication.
- If you are allergic to a particular herb, avoid it entirely or consult your physician before using it in any form (e.g., tea).

Tips for storing and preserving herbs

- Store herbs in a dry, cool place.
- Keep them out of direct sunlight.
- Do not store them in plastic bags or containers, as they are permeable to air and moisture. Instead, use glass jars with tight-fitting lids (sterilized with hot water if possible) or metal tins thoroughly cleaned with rubbing alcohol.

Herbal remedies for common ailments and health issues

Herbal remedies are an excellent way to treat many common disorders, including:

- Headaches and migraines
- Fatigue and low energy levels
- Digestive problems such as indigestion, gas, bloating, or constipation

Herbs can also help you maintain a healthy weight by improving your metabolism and digestion.

Herbalism's Roots in the Natural World

Herbalism is a practice that dates back to ancient times, and its roots can be traced back to our ancestors' relationship with nature. The natural world has always been essential to human culture; it shapes our language, art, music, and medicine. From Native tribes who used herbs for healing purposes or Chinese doctors who prescribed herbs alongside acupuncture treatments (known as "herb-acupuncture"), herbalism has always been an integral part of human life.

Herbs and People Have Always Been Connected

From the earliest days of civilization, herbs have played a role in human health and wellness. Many ancient cultures believed that certain herbs could help cure illness or even ward off death itself.

In this chapter, you'll learn about some of the most popular herbs used today--and how they became such an integral part of our daily lives.

The Roots of Herbalism Today

- You may be wondering how herbalism has become such a popular form of health and wellness today. Well, it all starts with the roots of herbalism itself.
- The first recorded use of herbs for medicinal purposes dates back to ancient Egypt, where physicians would prescribe certain plants to help them heal from various ailments. They also used these same herbs as an everyday part of their diet to promote good health and prevent disease from occurring at all.

Appreciating Nature's Healing Powers

It's time to take a closer look at some of the most popular herbs and their uses. We've got you covered if you want to learn more about nature's healing powers!

Herbs are a rich treasure of healing and wellness.

They have been used for thousands of years to support health, beauty, and well-being.

Herbs can be used as food, medicine, or cosmetic products. Some herbs are even considered sacred by many cultures around the world because they were revered for their healing properties long before modern medicine was developed.

The plants we call herbs can help heal many ailments and maintain optimal health.

Herbs are natural, medicinal plants that can treat a wide range of conditions. Herbs have been used for thousands of years, and many herbal remedies are still used today.

Herbs have been proven to help with a variety of health issues:

- Blood pressure (e.g., hawthorn)
- Depression (e.g., St John's wort)
- Diabetes (e.g., cinnamon)
- Digestive problems such as gas or bloating (e.g., peppermint)

Herbs have been used for centuries to treat and prevent health issues. Some herbs have anti-inflammatory properties, which can help to reduce pain and swelling.

- Turmeric is effective in reducing inflammation in the body. It's one of the main ingredients in curry powder, so if you love Indian food (and who doesn't?), try adding more turmeric into your diet instead of reaching for ibuprofen or aspirin!

Herbs can be used for childbirth and postpartum care, too.

Many of the herbs and essential oils mentioned above can also be used to support your pregnancy. For example, you may use lavender oil on your belly to help reduce swelling and promote circulation; peppermint oil in a bath to calm an upset stomach or help with nausea; sage tea as an aid in labor--the list goes on! And many of these same herbs will help with postpartum recovery as well: chamomile tea helps soothe sore breasts after breastfeeding; raspberry leaf tea promotes breast milk production and eases mastitis (breast inflammation); lemon balm tincture relieves cramping after birth; calendula salve treats cuts from cutting the cord or episiotomy stitches.

Herbs can be used to support healthy aging and combat the symptoms of menopause.

As you age, you may notice some changes in your body. Your hormones may be out of balance, and you may experience symptoms like hot flashes or night sweats. Herbs can help support healthy aging by balancing hormones and reducing these uncomfortable symptoms.

Hormonal imbalance is one of the main causes of menopause-related issues such as hot flashes and night sweats. Still, other factors can contribute to these problems, including stress levels, diet choices (including sugar consumption), exercise habits, and more. In addition to taking herbs that contain phytoestrogens (estrogen-like compounds found naturally in plants), such as black cohosh root extract or red clover flower extract, it's important to make changes in your everyday life so that you're living a healthier lifestyle overall so that all systems are functioning correctly!

Herbs can be helpful for digestive issues such as constipation and diarrhea.

Many herbs have a positive effect on the digestive system. These include aloe vera, ginger root, mint leaves, peppermint oil, and licorice root powder.

Natural remedies aren't just for hippies; they're scientifically proven methods to help your body heal itself.

You might think natural remedies are just for hippies, but they're scientifically proven methods to help your body heal itself.

Natural remedies can treat everything from colds and flu to anxiety, depression, and chronic conditions like eczema and psoriasis. They work because plants have healing properties that have been used for thousands of years--and many modern medicines are derived from them!

Herbalists believe that herbs have an intelligence within themselves that allows them to interact with the human body in a way beneficial for us when we use them properly. In other words: no matter what condition you're dealing with right now (or want to prevent), there's probably an herb out there that can help you feel better on some level.

Herbalism is the use of plants to promote health and wellness. Herbs can be used internally (tea, tincture) or externally (salve) to treat various ailments.

Herbalism has been practiced since antiquity in many cultures around the world, including China, India, Egypt, and Greece. In Europe, during medieval times, herbalists were often part of monasteries where they cultivated medicinal plants in their gardens for use by monks who were ill or injured.

Herbs are the original medicines, and they've been used for thousands of years to treat health conditions and promote wellness. They can be taken internally or applied externally, but they're generally considered safer and more effective when combined with other therapies.

Herbs stimulate or alter the body's natural systems, such as digestion or blood circulation. They're also known for their antioxidant properties, which protect against damage caused by free radicals (chemicals produced during normal cellular activity).

Herbs for your health and beauty

As you can see, herbs are a great way to achieve optimal health and beauty. But how do they work? Let's take a look at some of the most popular herbs used in today's world:

- Lavender: This flower has been used for centuries to treat depression, anxiety, insomnia and headaches. It also has antibacterial properties that make it useful for acne treatment.
- Chamomile: Chamomile tea is traditionally an effective sleep aid because it contains chamazulene, which helps reduce inflammation caused by stressors such as UV rays from sunlight.

169

What to Look for in a natural remedy

In order to make the most of your herbal remedies, it's important to understand what makes them so powerful. Here are some things to look for in a natural remedy:

- The herb should be grown organically with no pesticides or other chemicals added.
- The herbs should be harvested at their peak potency and dried at low temperatures (ideally less than 110 degrees F).

Use nature to help yourself be healthy.

Nature is a healer. It can help you feel better and live longer, but only if you are willing to learn how to use it. This book will teach you how to unlock the power of nature by using herbs for optimal health, wellness, and beauty.

You will discover:

- How herbs work with your body's natural systems to help heal from within
- The best way to prepare herbal remedies at home (and why it matters)
- A variety of ways that herbs can be used for specific conditions like acne or seasonal allergies

Herbal remedies have been around for centuries.

The ancient Egyptians used herbs to treat pain, infections, and other problems. Native herbs were known to use herbs in both their food and medicine. European herbalism dates back to at least 400 BC when Hippocrates prescribed them as part of his medical practice.

Herbs can be used to treat many conditions, including stress and anxiety.

- Stress is a major contributor to many health problems. It can cause inflammation in the body and increase cortisol levels (the stress hormone).
- Herbs known for their calming properties include chamomile, lavender, lemon balm, passionflower, and valerian root. These herbs have been used for centuries as natural remedies for stress relief because they contain compounds called essential oils that have calming effects on the body.

Herbal teas are easy to make and delicious.

You can use any combination of herbs in your tea, but try these classic combinations as a starting point:

- Chamomile and mint for relaxation
- Lemon balm or peppermint for digestion aid
- Rosemary and sage for cleansing the body

Many herbs are safe enough to use long-term.

Many herbs are safe enough to use long-term and can be just as effective as pharmaceutical drugs.

Herbs are often used instead of or alongside prescription medications because they're less likely to cause side effects. But many herbal products also have side effects, so it's important to research before using them.

You don't have to consult a doctor before taking herbal remedies. You may want to avoid doing so because they can be more likely than conventional drugs and supplements to interact with other medications or cause side effects. But if you want some advice on how best to use herbs and botanicals, talk with your doctor about your health goals and which herbs might help achieve them.

Herbs are powerful medicine!

Herbs can be used to treat a variety of health conditions, including:

- Mood disorders like depression and anxiety
- Digestive problems like constipation and diarrhea
- Skin conditions such as acne and eczema

Herbs are a powerful medicine! They can help you feel better and heal more quickly. Herbalism is an ancient practice used for centuries to treat ailments and maintain optimal health.

CONCLUSION

In conclusion, the "Herbal Remedies Natural Medicine Bible: [5 in 1]" is an excellent resource for anyone interested in natural medicine and the power of herbs and plants. With practical guides for growing and using healing herbs, preparing tinctures, essential oils, infusions, and antibiotics, this book provides information for those looking to take control of their health and well-being. Whether you're a seasoned herbalist or a beginner, this book has something to offer, and it's sure to become a go-to reference for years to come.

This book is a comprehensive resource for natural healing with detailed information on growing and using healing herbs and plants, preparing tinctures, essential oils, infusions, and antibiotics. Whether you are a beginner or an expert in herbal medicine, the practical guidance provided in this book will help you make informed decisions about your health and wellness. If you are looking for a reliable source of information on herbal remedies and natural medicine, this book is worth a read.

Made in the USA
Middletown, DE
14 June 2023

32641450R00097